the good medicine guide

Dr Vernon Coleman

the good medicine guide

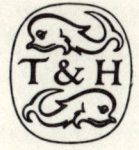

THAMES AND HUDSON

ISBN 0 500 01270 9

Filmset in Great Britain by Tameside Filmsetting Ltd,
Ashton-under-Lyne, Lancs.
Printed and bound in Great Britain by R. J. Acford,
Chichester, Sussex.

Contents

Contents

Preface 12

Health Care in Britain: an Introduction 13

The Professionals 29

General Practitioners 30

Family doctors: their basic responsibilities 30

GPs in private practice 30

GPs within the National Health Service 32

How the National Health Service GP is paid 38

The GP's premises 40

The treatment GPs provide 41

Sending the patient to a specialist 42

The primary care team 48

The average GP 52

The average doctor's working day 53

The average doctor's annual workload 57

Getting to see the doctor 58

Getting to see the doctor: points to remember 63

The consultation 64

What to tell the doctor 64

What to ask the doctor 65

FORMS AND CERTIFICATES USED BY THE GP 67

Choosing your doctor 70

Changing your doctor 73

Choosing or changing your doctor: points to remember 78

Patient participation 78

Ethical dilemmas 79

Making a complaint about a GP 98

Making a complaint to the FPC 100

Complaints about dentists, opticians and pharmacists 102

The five most important grounds for making a complaint about a GP to the Family Practitioner Committee 103

Making a complaint about a private GP 104

Legal action: when to sue 104

Going to the General Medical Council 105

Reasons for complaining about GPs 108

Reasons for not complaining about GPs 109

The top ten referrals most commonly made by GPs 45

The top ten consultants most commonly used by GPs 46

The top ten reasons for going to see a GP 62

Ten ways to keep your doctor sane 66

The top ten grumbles about GPs 99

Specialists **111**

Private specialists 111

Specialists within the National
Health Service 112

Getting the best out of a
specialist 115

Ethical dilemmas 117

Complaining about a specialist or any
other hospital doctor 118

A TO Z DIRECTORY OF
SPECIALISTS 122

Other Professionals **127**

A TO Z DIRECTORY OF OTHER
PROFESSIONALS 127

Private nurses 132

Alternative Professionals **133**

Why people use alternative medicine
and why they should take care when
they do 133

A TO Z GUIDE TO ALTERNATIVE
MEDICINE 135
QUALIFICATIONS TO LOOK FOR 140

The Institutions **141**

Health Service Hospitals, Homes and Clinics **142**

Hospitals 142

VD clinics 148

Involuntary admissions 148

Tips for getting admitted to an
NHS hospital if your problem is non-
urgent 149

Things they do to you in hospital and
why 150

Other institutions run by the state 153

*What to take with you when you go
into hospital* 152

Private Hospitals, Homes and Clinics **155**

Hospitals 155

Advantages of private hospital
treatment 156

Disadvantages of private hospital
treatment 157

Health farms and hydros 157

Nursing homes and rest homes 158

Advantages of nursing home care for
the elderly 160

Disadvantages of nursing home care
for the elderly 161

Points to remember when choosing a
private home for an old person 161

Screening clinics 163

Contents

The Organizations. 165

Statutory and Professional 166
A TO Z DIRECTORY OF STATUTORY AND PROFESSIONAL ORGANIZATIONS 166

Private and Voluntary 172
A TO Z DIRECTORY OF PRIVATE AND VOLUNTARY ORGANIZATIONS 174

Investigations and Tests 185
A TO Z DIRECTORY OF INVESTIGATIONS AND TESTS 186

Drugs and Treatments 195

Prescription Drugs 196

Obtaining a 'prescription only' drug 196

Categories of prescription drugs 197

The variety of products available 198

Branded or generic? 198

Drug efficiency 199

Patients' expectations 200

Placebos 200

How drugs should be taken ·201

Drug route 203

Storing medicines 204

To pay or not to pay 204

Repeat prescriptions 205

Drugs during pregnancy 208

Drugs during breastfeeding 208

Drugs for children 209

Unwanted effects of drugs 210

Sensitivity reactions 213

Drug interactions 214

Misuse of drugs 214

Poisoning 214

Tips for getting the best out of prescribed drugs 215

Reading a prescription 217

A sample prescription form 218

A DOG LATIN DICTIONARY 220

A TO Z OF COMMONLY PRESCRIBED DRUGS 222

HORMONE TREATMENTS 268

Oral contraceptives 269

Using the contraceptive pill: points to remember 270

Side effects with oral contraceptives 271

Vaccines 272

WHEN TO BE VACCINATED 275

Vitamins 278

A TO Z GLOSSARY OF PHARMACEUTICAL TERMS 280

A TO Z DIRECTORY OF MAJOR UK DRUG COMPANIES 285

The top ten prescription groups 207

Operative Procedures 295

OPERATIVE PROCEDURES: A TO Z DIRECTORY   295

Other Forms of Treatment 301

OTHER FORMS OF TREATMENT: A TO Z DIRECTORY   301

Home Care 303

Learning how to care at home   303   *Home screening: some major*
The Home Medicine Chest   307   *warning signs*   306

Health Insurance 309

Statutory Schemes 310

Rights and regulations   310   Non-contributory benefits   315
Contributory benefits   311

Private Schemes 318

The variety of schemes   Tips for choosing a private health
available   318   insurance scheme   320

Travelling at Home and Abroad 322

When Someone Dies: what has to be done 324

General Information 327

A TO Z DIRECTORY OF ABBREVIATIONS   Organ donors   337
COMMONLY USED IN MEDICINE   328   Medic Alert   337
A TO Z DIRECTORY OF QUALIFICATIONS   Guide to information sources   338
BY ABBREVIATION   334

Index 341

Preface

Professional medical care is big business these days. Thousands of millions of pounds and hundreds of thousands of people are devoted to the provision of health care facilities within both the government sponsored health service and the rapidly growing private health sector. The availability and quality of the service provided vary enormously according to the ways in which individual health care professionals interpret their own ethical responsibilities, their contractual commitments and their legal authority. Conflicting claims about the efficacy of contrasting forms of treatment, some of which are classified as orthodox and some of which are described as belonging to the school of alternative medicine, add to the variety of choice and contribute to the extent of the confusion that undoubtedly exists.

The sole purpose of this book is to enable the reader to understand and assess critically exactly what is offered by the various groups of health care professionals. We are all potential patients and potential consumers of health care, and we are, I believe, entitled to know how to make the best possible use of the facilities that are available, whether they are within or outside the National Health Service.

Sincerest thanks to Anne McDermid who was there at the beginning; to Jim Clayton who patiently helped in very many ways; to Eileen Reynolds who is one of the few people who can read my typing, let alone my handwriting; to the staff at Lisle Court who never complain; to Miss Edward and Mrs English at the Warwickshire Postgraduate Medical Centre Library who had to put up with many strange requests; to Peggy who got cramp queueing for social security leaflets; to my friends at Thames and Hudson whose expert hands eased the pains of labour; and to the countless others who contributed to the good bits but are quite entitled to blame me for the bad bits.   VC

Health Care in Britain: an Introduction

Before 1948, health care in Britain did not develop in any logical way or follow any organized medical philosophy.

Since the middle of the 19th century the medical profession had slowly acquired legal status, economic strength and social respectability, while the quality of medical care available had improved at varying speeds as scientists inside and outside the organized profession made important discoveries. Florence Nightingale's contribution both to the training of nurses and hospital planning had helped to revolutionize the standards of institutional care, and during the latter part of the 19th century a great many private and voluntary hospitals had been built, equipped, staffed and opened. At the beginning of the 20th century formal insurance schemes had been introduced to enable individual workers to protect themselves against the prospect of illness or accidental injuries affecting their capacity to work and requiring them to seek costly medical care.

But the progress made in these different areas had been patchy in quality and varied in availability. The standards in local authority hospitals varied enormously from one town to another and the type of medical care in prosperous areas differed tremendously from the type of care available in the slums and poorer country areas.

The National Health Service

It was in an attempt to eradicate these variations that the National Health Service was conceived, created and brought into being in 1948. The original aim was to provide free care, to improve the health of the people and eventually to reduce the demand for health care services simply by eradicating disease. The NHS took over all hospitals, convalescent homes and rehabilitation units and offered specialists full-time contracts as salaried employees. Family doctors were invited to sign contracts to provide services for patients in their area but they were allowed to remain self-employed, being paid by the new health service on a fee basis rather than a wage or salary basis.

The main advantage of the NHS was that it brought together all the services which had previously been under the control of independent organizations; this undoubtedly helped to improve the quality of care in those areas which had previously been without adequate services.

There were, however, administrative problems, mainly produced by the fact that the health service was still divided into three parts: that part which was under the care of the hospital boards and management committees; those individuals such as family doctors who were looked after by the local executive councils; and the type of care (such as ambulance services) provided by the local authorities themselves.

In an attempt to improve the coordination between these three supervising authorities, the politicians and senior administrators did a considerable amount of work on ways to reorganize the health service. The Labour government of 1968 published a Green Paper, which they amended in 1970, and the Conservative government which followed published a Consultative Document in 1971, and a White Paper in 1972. Eventually, in 1974, the National Health Service Reorganization Act came into being.

This new Act was intended to simplify the overall administration within the health service and to introduce a number of new channels through which health care professionals would be able to influence administrative decisions.

But, in practice, after 1974 the administrative machinery of the health service became almost unbelievably complex. Many writers have attempted to describe and explain exactly how the various parts of the machine fit together and what functions are served by the different departments, authorities and committees. Not one of the hundreds of books and articles about the health service which I have read has successfully accounted for existence of so many layers of administration.

I do not intend to add another incomprehensible chapter to the history of the health service but I will try and explain some the major pieces of the machine as it was left after 1974 and a is as I write.

Right at the top of the administrative hierarchy, of course, there is the Secretary of State for Social Services – an elected politician who may or may not know anything at all about health care. For the period of his appointment the Secretary of State is in total charge of the National Health Service, Personal Social Services and social security services. I will explain in a few moments the ways in which these three areas of responsibility differ.

The Secretary of State is, of course, assisted in his administrative duties by the Department of Health and Social Security, which itself consists of a large chunk of the civil service and which is mainly centred in offices at the Elephant and Castle in London. The DHSS, as the department is generally known, was formed in 1968 by a shotgun marriage which united the Ministry of Health and the Ministry of Social Security. The Secretary of State was originally known as the Secretary of State for Health and Social Services but somewhere along the line the word 'Health' was dropped from the title. The significance of this change is not known.

The DHSS does not itself provide or administer any practical health services but exists solely to ensure that other administrative groups provide such services. The DHSS is, however, responsible for organizing the provision of social security services, and the numerous local social security offices around the country are directly under the control of the central administration.

The number of full-time, highly paid administrators employed in the DHSS's central offices is naturally large, and understanding precisely what each member of this élite bureaucracy is next to impossible for a mere medical observer. For example, in one of its own explanatory publications the DHSS points out that the Chief Medical Adviser to Social Security Services has the status of a Deputy Chief Medical Officer in the DHSS, and the Deputy Chief Medical Adviser that of Senior Principal Medical Officer.

For all practical purposes the administrators employed at the DHSS's central office are beyond criticism, and when a Commons Select Committee dared to point out that the DHSS's long-term strategic planning and monitoring of health and social services was 'ineffective or non-existent' the DHSS immediately responded with a pungent attack on the Committee, pointing out that 'since they did not ask for information about the Department's machinery for strategic policy making they were not told about it.'

With the aid of the DHSS the Secretary of State is, as I have already explained, responsible for three distinct types of service. The social security section is the branch of the tree responsible for handing out pensions, sickness benefits and so on and in an average year in the early 1980s it will probably get through about £14,000 million: a substantial sum, which would work out at about £280 for every man, woman and child in the country if the administration of this department did not use up a large part of the total. Personal Social Services, the second branch, are handled by local authorities and consist of the provision of old people's homes, social workers, home helps and other non-medical aids. The third branch of the DHSS is the National Health Service, the branch with which this book is primarily concerned.

The highest tier in the NHS administration which has any practical responsibility and any real contact with sick people consists of the fourteen Regional Health Authorities which are responsible for long-term planning in their own Regions. They do have some responsibility for providing specialist facilities (such as blood transfusion services) and they have the authority to appoint consultants in all specialities, but their main task is to supervise the provision of health care services within their Region. There are no Regional Health Authorities in Wales, incidentally, and this tier of administration is missing entirely.

The Chairmen of the Regional Health Authorities receive a salary but the members who sit with them are unpaid. Each Authority has its own team of administrative officers which runs the Regional Health Authority on behalf of the members and with a wide range of advisory groups and committees of health professionals. There are quite a number of these committees. One Regional Health Authority was so dismayed when it discovered that its Medical Advisory Committee had itself got thirty-nine sub-committees that it set up another special committee to look into the number of committees in existence.

Beneath the Regional Health Authorities in the hierarchy there were until April 1982 ninety Area Health Authorities which usually had the same boundaries as local authority areas. The larger Area Health Authorities were divided into Districts and it is the Districts which today have a great deal of day-to-day responsibility for health care locally.

The District Management Teams which exist to look after the hospitals, health clinics, school health services and so on within each District within each Region are provided with the advice and information they need by groups of advisers and by the Community Health Councils.

There are about 200 Community Health Councils in England (there is one for every District) and they were formed to represent local community interests when it was realized that the administration had become so unwieldy that ordinary people were getting very little say in what the health service should or should not provide. The Community Health Councils were designed to provide the administrators with the view of the average man in the street with a broken leg. The members of the CHCs are nominated by the Regional Health Authorities, local voluntary organizations and local authorities. Naturally the Community Health Councils have administrative officers of their own. They cost some £4 million a year to run and a Bir-

Social services in England

(administration is different in Scotland, Wales and Northern Ireland)

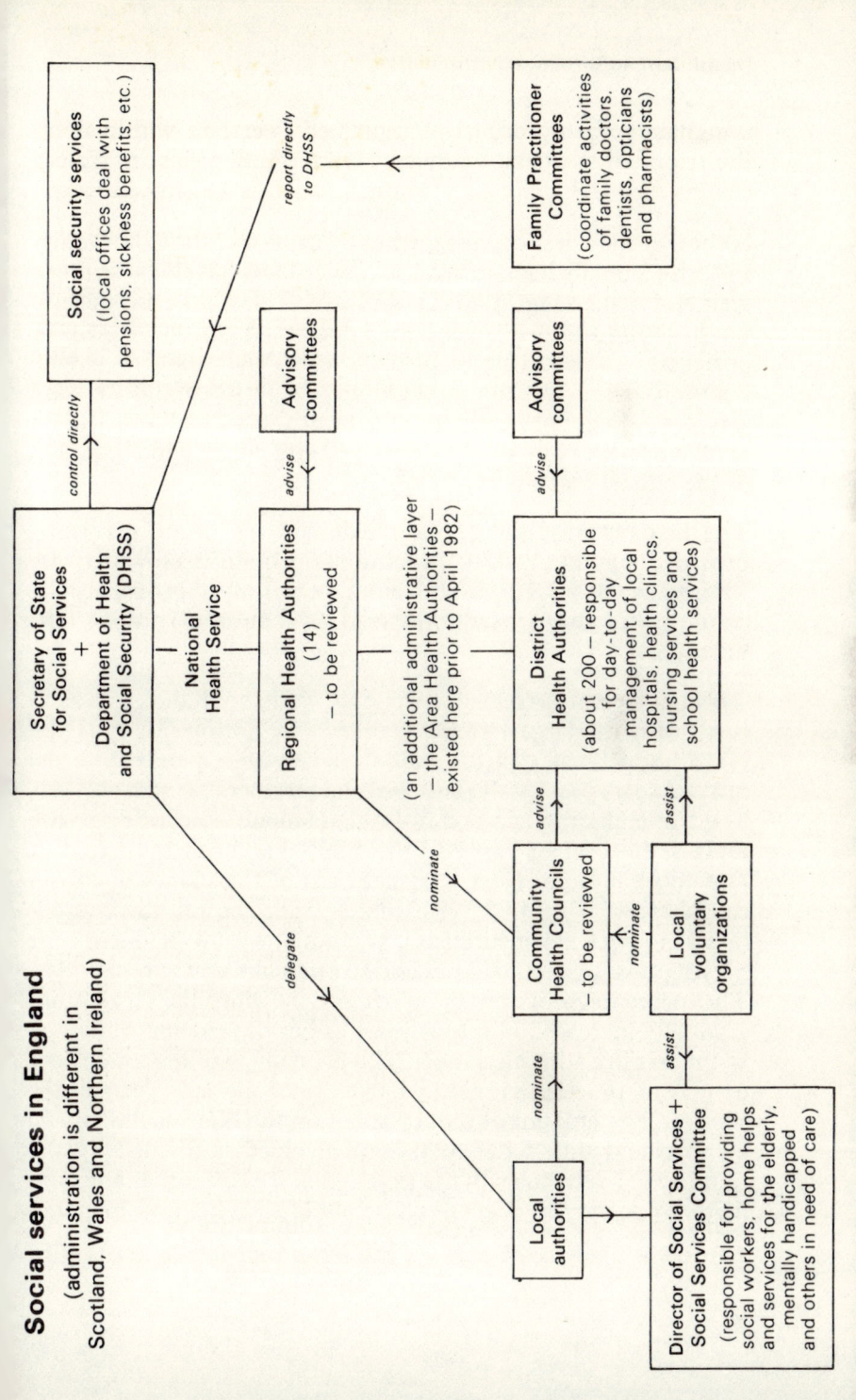

Secretary of State for Social Services + Department of Health and Social Security (DHSS)

control directly → **Social security services** (local offices deal with pensions, sickness benefits, etc.)

report directly to DHSS

National Health Service

Regional Health Authorities (14) – to be reviewed — *advise* — **Advisory committees**

(an additional administrative layer – the Area Health Authorities – existed here prior to April 1982)

District Health Authorities (about 200 – responsible for day-to-day management of local hospitals, health clinics, nursing services and school health services) — *advise* — **Advisory committees**

Family Practitioner Committees (coordinate activities of family doctors, dentists, opticians and pharmacists)

nominate → **Community Health Councils** – to be reviewed — *advise*

Local voluntary organizations — *assist* — *nominate*

delegate → **Local authorities**

nominate → **Director of Social Services + Social Services Committee** (responsible for providing social workers, home helps and services for the elderly, mentally handicapped and others in need of care) — *assist*

mingham surgeon recently complained that they simply sit on the fringe of the health service waiting for someone to drop a clanger.

Although the District Management Teams and the Community Health Councils have jurisdiction over local hospitals, and can visit and make suggestions about the way they are run, they do not have any authority over family doctors, dentists, chemists or opticians. In fact, these 'primary care' practitioners – who between them actually provide the majority of health care services – do not fit neatly into the health service administration at all since they are all self-employed and entirely independent of the official machinery.

The link between these individuals and the health service is provided by the Family Practitioner Committees which are advised and provided with information by a number of specialist committees, and are administered by teams of professional bureaucrats.

This massive organization costs over £10,000 million a year to run and is the largest single employer in Europe. In 1981 the NHS budget was £13,300 million (a rise of 55 per cent on the bill two years previously) and the total number of employees was listed as including 800,000 in England alone. According to the DHSS the cost of running the NHS has been estimated at £20,000 a minute. Nearly 90 per cent of the money spent on the National Health Service comes from central government taxation; national insurance contributions, and payments for prescriptions, dental charges and so on, make up the remainder. The percentage of money spent on the hospital service has gradually increased in recent years as has the amount of money spent on pure administration. The percentage of the total spent on general practice has nearly halved since the early years of the service. The amount of money spent on the NHS is difficult to comprehend but if the total sum involved is divided by the number of individuals in the population it is clear that approximately £200 a year is spent on behalf of each man, woman and child.

It is not only the cost and complexity of the administrative hierarchy that causes doubts about the effectiveness and efficiency of the National Health Service. There is a considerable amount of valid statistical evidence to support the contention that the British health service does not provide good value for money.

Most important of all the statistics are those which show the mortality and morbidity rates in Britain compared with other Western European countries. Sadly these show that life expectation in Britain does not seem to be benefiting from the care available and that the British infant mortality rate (a statistic commonly used to enable observers to judge the effectiveness of a country's health care facilities) is among the worst in the western world.

Almost equally depressing are those statistics which show that there are now some 650,000 people on hospital waiting lists in Britain, many of whom will have to wait years before they can be admitted and some of whom will die before they can obtain the treatment to which they may have thought themselves entitled. The government's own figures also show that although expenditure on the health service has consistently risen faster than inflation the number of people taking time off work through sickness is increasing. And while some administrators work in luxurious offices a large number of hospitals in use in Britain were built before the beginning of this century. Two-thirds of the beds available in British hospitals today are in those hospitals which were built in the 19th century by private organizations and there are fewer beds altogether available today than there were when the NHS was founded in 1948. Compared with other countries in the European Economic Community Britain has dismally few hospital beds available. The average number of beds per 1000 people in the EEC is 10.3. In Britain the average number of beds per 1000 people is 8.1.

Although the NHS was originally founded to iron out the inequalities in medical care there is considerable evidence to suggest that many of those inequalities have still not been dealt with. Twice as many babies of unskilled parents die as do babies of more affluent classes and long-standing illness is much more common among unskilled workers than it is among the professional classes. Waiting lists in different parts of the country vary enormously and while in pleasant suburbs and pretty country areas general practitioners have relatively few patients to look after, family doctors working in the less pleasant parts of big cities are responsible for the health care of up to twice as many patients. The time they can spend on each consultation is almost inevitably halved.

Wastage in the health service is horrifying. Because there are few checks on overall spending and no incentive to save money, millions of pounds are wasted annually on unnecessary tests, esoteric research, pointless conferences, thoughtless prescribing, and silly habits such as switching hospital heating on and off according to specified dates rather than according to the weather. This last point may produce a wry smile but many large hospitals spend £1½ million a year on fuel and bills could in many cases be halved without difficulty or inconvenience to patients or staff.

But there are no incentives for savings to be made. If for any reason the amount of money allocated to a particular department is not used up within a financial year then the amount of money allocated the following year will be reduced accordingly. The result of this is that towards the end of each financial year administrators and advisory committees all over the country are busy working out ways to get rid of surplus money – often by spending it on equipment that is not really needed.

Before the 1974 reorganization, hospital matrons had considerable power within their own empires. They were responsible for maintaining standards of nursing care, cleanliness and discipline and by and large they did their jobs exceptionally well. Partly because of the changes which resulted from the 1974 reorganization and partly as a result of yet another report which recommended changes in the structure of the nursing profession the hospital matron no longer exists. Today we have a bureaucracy within a bureaucracy and in each hospital there are several layers of nursing officers given the responsibility for maintaining nursing standards. Out of 400,000 nurses in England and Wales, nearly one in four (all of them good, well-trained nurses) has no direct responsibility for or contact with patients. There are nine grades of nursing administrator above the level of ward sister. And yet while the size of the nursing bureaucracy has risen the extent of their shared responsibility has fallen. Today nurses no longer have responsibility for anything other than simple practical nursing chores. They have no brief to look after their patients in anything other than a purely clinical way. And to deal with those other duties the hospitals have had to employ many more administrators. One hospital group, for example, is said to employ a full-time curtain manager to do nothing else but look after curtains. During the last few years the number of clerks and administrators working in the NHS has risen far faster than the number of doctors or working nurses.

The ambulance service costs over £150 million a year and the number of people using ambulances to get to and from hospitals has risen steadily during the lifetime of the National Health Service. But less than 10 per cent of all journeys involve accident victims or emergency admissions. The majority of those using the ambulance service could travel by car or public transport. Ambulances are used because they are free and convenient and because there is no incentive for anyone to limit their availability. In fact the cost of running an ambulance is so high that some health authorities actually use taxis to ferry patients. One NHS spokesman told me that during a recent ambulance strike the great majority of patients booked to travel to hospital by ambulance still managed to make their own way to their out-patient appointments.

Money is spent in huge quantities on research projects which promise little in the way of useful results but a great deal in the way of kudos for those responsible. Britain leads the way in test tube babies, fallopian tube transplantation, pelvic arteriography, amniocentesis, ultrasound, computerized tomograms and even some aspects of transplantation and yet, as we have seen, we have one of the worst infant mortality rates in the western world, and a man with an operable cancer may have to go on a waiting list before his condition can be properly investigated or treated. If you have porphyria then you will get the best treatment in the world but if you are old, depressed or arthritic then you will get treated worse in Britain than just about anywhere else. The man who pays the piper does not necessarily have the right to choose all the tunes, but surely he has the right to listen to the music occasionally.

None of these facts is unrecognized by the professional administrators at the DHSS in London and few there would argue with the facts I have listed or the interpretation I have put on them. Unfortunately, the administrators who run the National Health Service have no more idea about how to stop the wastage, how to improve the quality of care or how to iron out the inequalities than anyone else. Nor do any of the government's numerous advisers seem to have any enthusiasm for change.

Since the 1974 reorganization successive governments have continued to search for answers to the problems which undoubtedly exist. In 1979, for example, just under £1 million was spent on a Royal Commission on the National Health Service. The Commission found, among other things, that one-fifth of surgical patients had been on the waiting list for more than two years, but it nevertheless decided that on the whole health workers paint too gloomy a picture of the NHS and it concluded with a number of suggestions for improvements. These included such shattering philosophical developments as the proposal that the Scottish system for recording information about the dental treatment of children should be adopted in the rest of the UK. The Commission also suggested that a select committee on the NHS should be set up, but when that select committee was set up and it reported that the DHSS had done nowhere near enough planning for the future of the health service the government, advised by the DHSS, rejected the complaint.

Occasionally brave attempts have been made to do something about the uneven distribution of facilities within the health service and about the wastage that saps its strength. For example, one British minister recently pointed out that the health service cannot possibly attend to all human ills and suggested that people with minor ailments should treat themselves in order to reduce pressure on the NHS. His seemingly sensible and well-intentioned plea was not well received. The *Daily Mirror*, for example, which has on several occasions published reports drawing attention to the inadequacies of the health service, used the statement as the basis for a front-page story headlined 'Minister attacks the sick'.

Towards the end of 1980, in an attempt to cut administrative costs, it was announced that the Area Health Authorities would be scrapped in 1982 and that this would cut the £300 million-a-year management and administration cost by 10 per cent. An official statement pointed out that after six years' experience of the 1974 reforms the DHSS had come to the conclusion that there was no need for Area Health Authorities to interfere between District Management Teams and Regional Health Authorities.

Inevitably, perhaps, the suggestion produced a furore among administrators and even seemed to attract disapproval from many public commentators, who all pointed out that the planned changes seemed extremely unlikely to reduce the real cost of the service or to improve the quality of the service for patients. It will at some future date be easy enough to produce accounts which show that the deletion of a tier of administration has saved money, but, as long as such savings come out of as yet unplanned budgets and so can be lost amidst changes due to inflation, the savings will be meaningless.

There are not, of course, any simple solutions to the problems which afflict the National Health Service. The original dream that free care for all would mean good health for all and the abolition of disease has become a nightmare for many and we need to think again about our needs and expectations.

Medical science has developed in many different ways during the last century and a half and the social and scientific advances which have preceded, accompanied, and sometimes followed those developments have meant that the relationship of health care to life, living conditions and general expectations must have changed.

We need to re-evaluate our expectations, learn to differentiate between caring and curing, and make fundamental decisions about whether or not all available forms of treatment are to be made available to all patients in need, about how we are going to evaluate competing therapies or diagnostic aids, about what priorities we are going to select, about the value of preventive medicine in future health programmes, about the extent to which qualified personnel can delegate work, about the responsibilities of the health care services, about the relative values of primary care and hospital care, and about what we want from our researchers. There are ethical, economic, social and philosophical dilemmas which must be solved before the NHS can ever be reorganized effectively or efficiently and messing about with an admittedly chaotic administration will not answer any of these questions.

Private health care

It is not my aim in this book to try to deal with these questions or to make proposals for the improvement of the existing health service. The aim of *The Good Medicine Guide* is to enable you to make the best possible use of the health care facilities which exist at the moment in Britain.

That aim would not be fulfilled if I ignored the rapidly growing and immensely important facilities made available by the many private health care organizations, institutions and associations in Britain.

Many of the proponents of private health care argue that one of the major problems with the NHS is the fact that the relationship between doctor and patient has been damaged by the intervention of a third party, the state, which pays the doctor on behalf of the patient and which creates the rules surrounding the relationship.

Only where the patient and the doctor have a direct relationship can the quality of the service provided meet the necessary standards, the argument continues. Patients want to have time to talk to their doctor, they want to be able to choose when any necessary operation is performed, they do not want to wait for long periods of time, they want to know exactly who will perform necessary surgical procedures and they want to be assured of some continuity of care. More than anything else, say those who advocate private medical care, people want to keep away from the National Health Service since they consider it to be an avoidable health risk.

It is certainly true that the last few years have seen a tremendous rise in the demand for private medical services. In 1979 alone 174,000 new subscribers joined the three main insurance companies, British United Provident Association (BUPA), Private Patients Plan (PPP) and Western Provident Association (WPA), and the people carrying insurance entitling them to private medical care were, between them, paying £124 million in subscriptions to the nine leading provident associations. These insured individuals made up only about half of the total numbers seeking private care and by 1980 there were 150 private hospitals in Britain with full operating theatre facilities, 1000 registered nursing homes and 2000 registered private rest homes.

At the beginning of 1981 the largest two organizations, BUPA and PPP, said that during 1980 the numbers of their subscribers had risen by 25 per cent despite the effects of the recession. BUPA alone had a net increase of nearly 300,000 subscribers during the year, bringing its total number of paying members to 1,250,000. With dependants, that gave BUPA alone responsibility for the private medical care of almost 3 million people. Whether you agree with it as a principle or not you have to accept that today private medical care is no longer a fringe medical activity, but does provide a major alternative to the care provided in Britain through the National Health Service.

At the same time as there has been an increase in the number of orthodox, allopathic practitioners providing private medical care, there has also been a tremendous increase in the number of practitioners offering alternative forms of care. Some of these alternatives are discussed on pp. 133–39.

The following sections are devoted to a simple, straightforward, factual analysis of the services available through the National Health Service and through the various private practitioners, private hospitals and medical insurance companies, whether they be representative of the organized, traditional British medical profession or of one or other of the many groups offering forms of medical care.

The Professionals

☐ *General Practitioners*

☐ *Specialists*

☐ *Other Professionals*

☐ *Alternative Professionals*

□ General Practitioners

Family doctors: their basic responsibilities

The family doctor or general medical practitioner has two main functions.

First, he is expected to provide medical care for those illnesses and symptoms that cannot be dealt with effectively at home without professional attention. And, second, he is expected to know when his own capacity to provide useful assistance is no longer enough. He must know when to seek more specialist help, and he must know where to find that help and how to make the best use of whatever specialist facilities may be available.

The second function is, if anything, more important than the first, for the general practitioner who does not know the limits of his own knowledge and capabilities is a threat to his patients.

The importance of the role played by the family doctor in 20th-century medicine can be judged from the fact that, in the countries where family doctoring has long been a forgotten branch of the profession, there has in recent years been a strong revival in the demand for doctors who can link the varying skills offered by individual specialists, and who can explain the alternatives to their patients. Paradoxically, as the number of medical specialities has grown, so has the demand and need for general practitioners.

There are two main ways in which general medical care may be provided in Britain: through the health service and privately.

GPs in private practice

Although the majority of general practitioners in Britain work with the National Health Service and spend their time wholly or mainly looking after health service patients, there are a few private GPs, mostly working in large towns and cities, who operate entirely independently of the NHS.

It is, I think, important to point out here that the laws in Britain do not prevent anyone from practising as a doctor. It is perfectly legal for any individual to set up in practice as a physician, surgeon or general practitioner and to offer advice and help without having any qualifications at all. It is only *illegal* to do this if, in addition, the individual unjustifiably claims to be a registered medical practitioner. Although the unregistered practitioner may be liable to charges of assault if he practises with no training and no licence, and could find himself facing charges in the civil courts, there is nothing in British law to prevent any unqualified practitioner from opening a surgery or office.

Registered medical practitioners, however, whether they are in health service practice or in private practice must have qualifications which have been recognized by the General Medical Council. So the individual patient looking for an orthodox, qualified private practitioner can expect to find evidence of the same qualifications as the patient seeking an NHS practitioner (see pp. 334 ff.).

A patient who opts to see a private practitioner does not have to make any commitment to that doctor, although there are some practitioners in private practice who offer annual subscriptions to their patients. The patient pays a fixed sum for a year's medical care and may then have to pay an additional sum for each consultation, visit and prescription. Registered medical practitioners in private practice can sign some official certificates but they are not allowed to use health service prescription pads. Some private family doctors do refer patients to specialists in health service hospitals, but the majority of practitioners in private practice refer patients requiring consultant care to a specialist who is also in private practice.

Incidentally, the majority of provident insurance companies (such as BUPA) do not provide facilities for their members to be seen by private general practitioners.

Although most private medical practitioners work independently there are certain organizations offering forms of private care which need to be mentioned.

'Dial a doctor'

In London, for example, there is now an organization called Medicover, known as the 'dial a doctor' service. For a fixed annual sum subscribers are guaranteed a visit from a registered medical practitioner at any time they ring. An additional sum has to be paid for each visit.

Private screening clinics

In addition there are now a number of private screening clinics available in Britain. For a fixed sum, patients – who can be seen even if they are registered with a health service practitioner – will receive a full medical check-up.

Whether screening programmes are effective (in so far as the check-up only tells the patient whether or not any pathology has been found at the time of examination) is a question still subject to considerable debate (see pp. 163–64). Many authorities in the field of preventive medicine now feel that disease can be prevented more effectively by teaching patients how to watch out for early signs of impending illness than by performing annual medical check-ups, which are costly in terms of equipment and skilled workers, and relatively inefficient in terms of picking up early signs of disease. (See pp. 303 ff. for home screening suggestions.)

GPs within the National Health Service

The first and most important point about general practitioners within the National Health Service is that they are not directly employed by the state (even though they are paid by it) in the same way that doctors working in hospitals or for local authorities are directly employed.

As a result of historical events which are not really relevant to this book (but which can easily be investigated by those with a mind to do so) GPs have remained independent and self-employed during the whole period of the health service. The state may have come between doctors and patients and may have been responsible for drawing up the rules about work conditions, pay, and all other aspects of the relationship, but as I described in the Introduction family doctors do not fit neatly into the bureaucratic hierarchy.

As far as the administration of the health service is concerned the fact that GPs are self-employed is undoubtedly a disadvantage. It means that the health service mandarins, instead of having to deal with a single body of employed workers with specific responsibilities, have to deal with a small army of individuals tied together loosely by the same general rules and regulations but allowed considerably more freedom than any other group within the health service.

As far as the family doctors themselves are concerned there are advantages and disadvantages in remaining self-employed. In exchange for a certain amount of personal and professional freedom, the GP must agree to contractual commitments which no salaried employee would be expected to consider, let alone tolerate. I will describe what I mean by this a little later on.

There are advantages and disadvantages for patients too. One of the main disadvantages is that there are many administrative contrasts between practices in various parts of the country. Because GPs are self-employed and because most of them own their own premises there are tremendous differences between the types of care available within the NHS framework.

To counteract these advantages, however, there are certain advantages, the main one being that the self-employed GP is able to provide those patients for whom he is responsible with care and attention which is not affected by responsibility to any higher authority. What this means in practice is that the GP is free to nag and worry at any part of the health service administration which seems to be failing any patient at any time. A GP who was directly employed and who had a specific role and status within the bureaucracy would be far less able to provide his patients with the sort of independent advice and assistance that they often need.

Terms of Service

Each general practitioner in Britain with a list of NHS patients is known as a 'principal', and when taking on a list, or obtaining the right to acquire one, each doctor has to sign a contract with the local Family Practitioner Committee. It is this contract which outlines the responsibilities of GPs to their health service patients.

The Terms of Service, which are the basis of the doctor's contract, are complex, but the most important inclusions are obviously those which describe precisely what the GP's responsibilities are to be.

It is, for example, laid down that the GP shall 'render to his patients all necessary and appropriate personal medical services of the type usually provided by general medical practitioners' and that 'he shall do so at his practice premises, or, if the condition of the patient so requires, elsewhere in his practice area.' The GP is also contractually bound to make arrangements for referring his patients as may be necessary to any of the other services provided within the NHS.

Unless prevented from doing so by an emergency a family doctor must attend and treat any patient who visits his surgery during the hours at which he has said that he will be there. The only exception to this is when a patient attends without an appointment when an appointment system is in operation. If that is the case, the doctor can refuse to treat the patient as long as the patient's health will not be jeopardized and, of course, as long as the patient is offered an appointment for some future date. The Terms of Service include a clause which states that the doctor should take all reasonable steps to ensure that a patient is not turned away by a receptionist.

There are no limitations on these responsibilities and therefore the GP is contractually committed to provide care for 24 hours a day on every day of the year. That contract commitment can only be revoked if the doctor's contract is formally ended by either the Family Practitioner Committee or the doctor concerned.

There are still some single-handed GPs who do provide 24-hour-a-day cover for all their patients and who simply hire a locum for their two weeks' annual holiday. But most family doctors operate rota systems with partners or other local practitioners and will share the responsibility of looking after each other's patients. A number of GPs reduce their 'out of hours' commitments even further by using deputizing services to answer night and emergency calls. The deputizing services, some of which are non-profit-making and some of which are commercial organizations, employ doctors on a part- or full-time basis. Incidentally, the doctor's responsibility under his contract does not end when a locum or deputy is employed and, in theory at least, a GP who is himself ill in hospital or abroad on holiday is still responsible for his patients and for providing them with medical care. If no locum can be found to cover for a sick practitioner the doctor must rise from his sick bed (and many have done so), and if the locum makes a mistake it is the GP's responsibility and he who must respond to any complaint. You will now perhaps see what I meant when I claimed that the GP's self-employed status leaves him with responsibilities which no salaried employee would tolerate.

It is perhaps hardly surprising that the number of GPs committing suicide, turning to alcohol or requiring treatment for serious depression is higher than for most other groups of workers. By and large GPs do not live long lives.

Variations in the service provided by GPs

When we think of the National Health Service most of us think of it as being one mammoth organization providing identical facilities throughout the country. The principle of the scheme is, after all, that whatever you earn and wherever you live you will get exactly the same type of medical care as everyone else. If you have a duodenal ulcer and live in Darlington you should get the same type of care as if you have a duodenal ulcer and live in Truro. Unfortunately, of course, it isn't quite like that. Even allowing for the fact that the NHS is operated by human beings whose skills, aptitudes, interests and so on vary, there are some astonishing, quite fundamental differences in the services provided.

Just as there are differences in the quantity and quality of hospital facilities available, so there are enormous differences in the quality of general practitioner services provided in different areas. The most important single factor that affects the quality of service available in any one area must be the number of patients cared for by each GP. There is no fixed pattern of doctor shortages and indeed within one county boundary there may well be doctors with less than 2000 patients on their lists and doctors with over 3000 patients on their lists. Since every GP can only work for so many hours in the day the patients who are on the list with 3000 other people must see less of their doctor.

Since the inception of the National Health Service the government has attempted to move GPs from the well-serviced areas to the areas which are short of GPs. In practice this has not been easy since the poorly doctored areas tend to be unattractive parts of large cities where working conditions are miserable and schooling and social facilities poor.

Areas have been classified according to the size of the average lists in each area. The most poorly serviced areas are known as Designated areas and these are the places where in theory doctors have, on average, more than 3000 patients on their lists.

In an attempt to steer doctors towards the Designated areas many rules and regulations have been set up to act as deterrents and incentives. For example, a doctor will receive a special payment if he works in a Designated area and intends dealing (as most doctors do) with National Health Service patients. In practice these rules have been ineffective and the areas which were short of doctors twenty years ago are short of doctors today. There is still a grave shortage of general practitioners in parts of the Midlands and the north and a comparative excess in some of the choicer areas of the south. Doctors, having personal and family responsibilities and ties, will, like everyone else, usually end up working where they have friends, contacts or relatives.

Abuses

The general practitioner's contract commitments unfortunately provide ample opportunity for abuse by both doctors and patients.

For example, GPs can earn considerable amounts of money for very small amounts of work if they are prepared to offer their patients the minimum service required by the NHS. It is possible for a GP with a large number of patients on his list to accept the money for looking after those patients but to pass on his responsibilities regularly to hospital staff, referring almost all the patients he sees to hospital consultants and doing little real medical work himself. The GP without good intentions may consider his patients nothing more than an administrative nuisance; he may be rude to them and he may fail to provide them with support, explanations or advice. Nevertheless, the rules allow him to continue to practise in this way without being disciplined.

On the other hand, there are many opportunities for patients to abuse the system too. Patients can in turn be rude, over-demanding and aggressive. They can cause a thoughtful and considerate practitioner much heartache by unjustifiably complaining about him to the Family Practitioner Committee; they can expect an amount of attention that would mean the practitioner could retain a list of no more than a hundred patients; and they may consider themselves at war with their practitioner, just as he may feel he is at war with them. The truth is, of course, that the family doctor service in the NHS depends on trust and goodwill from both sides.

Where that trust and goodwill exist there is little doubt in my mind that the family doctor service can provide patients with an enormously important type of care. It is, after all, only a family doctor who can acquire the extent and depth of medical and social knowledge that will enable an individual patient to be treated as a human being, a member of a family group and of a community, rather than simply as a collection of tissues and organs exhibiting some temporary pathology.

How the National Health Service GP is paid

As a self-employed practitioner the NHS GP is paid on a fee basis rather than on a salary or wage basis. The actual way in which a practitioner's aggregate income is made up is so complex that even GPs themselves frequently admit that they do not completely understand all the variations and possibilities.

The basic fee is the payment made by the government for each patient on the doctor's list. This is called a Capitation Fee and it amounts to several pounds a head for each year's care. As I write, the standard Capitation Fee for a patient under the age of 65 is £4.65; the fee for a patient between the ages of 65 and 74 is £6.05; and the fee for a patient over the age of 75 is £7.45. The additional payments for older patients are in recognition of the fact that older patients usually need more medical attention than younger patients.

In addition to these fees the GP will receive an annual payment simply for being in practice with the NHS. This is called a Basic Practice Allowance and it varies according to the area in which the doctor is practising, the number of years he has been in practice and whether or not he employs an assistant.

That is just the very beginning. There are in addition special fees for providing contraceptive advice and maternity advice, for performing vaccinations, for treating temporary residents, for attending patients at night, for performing cervical cytology tests, for having a trainee in the practice and for an enormous variety of other services.

Doctors working in their own premises (as most do) are entitled to claim rent allowances, rate rebates and a proportion of the money they must spend on hiring receptionists, nurses and other staff members. General practitioners do not receive any financial help towards the cost of equipment, telephones, heating and light, petrol, or drugs they need to use when they are visiting patients in an emergency.

The way in which fees are allocated does not always seem entirely logical. For example, a doctor can theoretically claim three separate fees if he gives a child separate vaccinations for whooping cough, tetanus and diphtheria, or just one fee payment if he gives the child the same immunizations in a single jab. The doctor who provides his patients with X-ray facilities or urine testing facilities must pay for the equipment and technical staff out of his own pocket, whereas the GP who does not provide these facilities is entitled to use hospital facilities without charge. A doctor who works in a group practice with two other GPs will receive an additional payment of several hundred pounds a year for simply being a member of a group.

All things considered, NHS payments do not add anything to the quality of care provided, since they reward the doctor who has a large list and does no tests of his own far better than the doctor with a small list who does much of his own diagnostic work.

Nearly all full-time NHS general practitioners have an additional income from other sources. Signing certificates often brings in additional sums since the GP is only bound by law to provide a limited number of certificates (such as a death certificate and a national insurance sick note) without charge. In addition a number of GPs do work as clinical assistants in local hospitals, as industrial medical officers, as police surgeons, as prison medical officers or as medical examiners for insurance companies.

A relatively small number of GPs have private patients. NHS general practitioners are allowed to see patients privately but no patient can be half health service patient and half private patient. In other words a private patient must pay for all the treatment he receives – and that includes drugs provided on prescription.

The GP's premises

The traditional family doctor used to practise in his own home. In some the dining room table would be cleared so that the room could be used as a patients' waiting room.

Today, relatively few doctors practise in their own homes, although the majority still practise in premises which they themselves own. Some doctors work in converted houses while others work in specially built medical centres.

A few years ago it was official government policy to encourage general practitioners to work in publicly owned 'health centres'. The idea was that, together with family doctors, there would be local nurses, chiropodists, dentists and all sorts of other professionals offering services. A few hundred health centres have been built and a relatively small percentage of family doctors do work in such centres but the scheme has never really become a great success. One problem has been simply finding the money – it is cheaper for the government if GPs buy their own premises even if they then claim a special rent allowance back from the government. A more important problem, however, is the fear of working in an officially owned centre. Since they are self-employed many GPs feel that they will be extremely vulnerable if they work in premises they do not own. The argument is that the GP who works in premises he owns can always resign from the NHS and see only private patients.

Since neither the administrators nor the GPs themselves are very keen on health centres it is hardly surprising that there are not many of them.

The treatment GPs provide

The majority of consultations between a general practitioner and a patient end with the former providing the latter with a prescription. There is a strong historical reason for the fact that so many meetings end with a prescription: several centuries ago members of the Society of Apothecaries (the forerunners of today's GPs) were not allowed to charge patients for advice but only for providing drugs. This was a result of effective political pressure applied by the College of Physicians and it meant that apothecaries always ended a consultation with a prescription.

Most general practitioners only provide their patients with actual drug supplies in an emergency (doctors carry emergency supplies of a small number of basic medicines – they must either buy these supplies themselves or obtain them from a kindly drug company representative), but a small number of family doctors who practise in rural areas do their own dispensing, providing the patient directly with a supply of the prescribed medicine.

The other services provided by family doctors vary from practice to practice. Nearly all GPs will syringe ears, change dressings, remove stitches and do other simple chores (or they will have a nurse who will do these tasks), but relatively few modern GPs will perform minor surgery or indeed carry out any procedure expensive in terms of equipment or time. The reason for this is simple: the GP does not receive a fee for providing treatment facilities and would be operating at a financial loss if he were to do so. A very small number of GPs have direct access to hospital beds in cottage hospitals or general practitioner hospitals. These beds are usually filled by patients requiring nursing care during convalescence.

A small, and declining, number of GPs still take full responsibility for their pregnant patients. They provide ante-natal clinics and attend all their expectant patients during labour. These doctors may have access to beds in special labour wards in a local maternity hospital or the maternity wing of a general hospital.

The majority of GPs, however, provide a limited service for their pregnant patients. They will provide ante-natal care, either at special clinics usually held in the surgery or at ordinary surgery sessions, but they will hand over care during labour to a local obstetrician. Unlike GPs who provide comprehensive care for their pregnant patients doctors in this second, larger, group are usually unwilling to allow their patients to have their babies at home. Some argue that confinement in hospital is safer for both mother and baby while others admit that they do not consider themselves technically competent to provide a full range of obstetric services in the home.

(Drug treatments and prescribing habits are discussed on pp. 196ff.)

Sending the patient to a specialist

The general practitioner's job does not only involve providing patients with treatment. The family doctor also has a responsibility to ensure that his patients are referred to the appropriate specialist agencies when additional help is required. The GP who does not make the appropriate referrals is in fact in breach of his contract with the local Family Practitioner Committee.

Naturally many problems cannot be dealt with effectively or safely by the family doctor and a specialist's advice must be sought – either because only the specialist has the necessary knowledge, or because only he has access to the diagnostic equipment required, or because only he has access to the equipment and facilities required to perform a technical procedure (such as a surgical operation) and the skill to perform it.

Tests

The simplest referrals are those which involve sending the patient along for specialist tests. In an ideal world all general practitioners would be equipped with microscopes, electro-cardiograms, X-ray machines and small laboratories. The availability of such facilities would improve the quality of service provided by family doctors and would reduce the pressure on the hospital service. Unfortunately, the present method of paying general practitioners pretty well discourages the majority of GPs from providing all these facilities. And so patients must be sent to local hospitals. The range of tests available to GPs varies from area to area but a description of most of the tests commonly performed can be found on pp. 186–94.

Emergencies

Referrals to the hospital system fall into two main categories. First, and most important, there are the emergency referrals. For example, a patient may have acute abdominal pains which suggest a diagnosis of appendicitis. The procedures involved in making such an emergency referral vary from one part of the country to another. In London there is an Emergency Bed Service which provides general practitioners with up-to-date information about the availability of hospital beds. In many other parts of the country, however, the general practitioner must simply telephone hospital after hospital, speaking to a junior hospital doctor or administrator in each establishment, until he finds a hospital with a vacant bed. Then he must persuade the hospital doctor responsible for admitting new patients to accept the admission. Obviously no hospital doctor is going to refuse to admit a genuine emergency.

Other referrals

Less dramatic are those referrals that are not emergencies (though they may still be fairly urgent). In these cases the general practitioner or one of his administrative representatives will telephone or write to a specific, named local specialist and obtain an out-patient appointment. If the problem is obviously not an urgent one (a bad varicose vein, for example, is not an urgent problem) then the referring practitioner will simply ask for a straightforward appointment. If, however, the problem needs attention without delay then the GP will make this point clear in his letter of referral. When making up the appointment lists for his out-patient clinics the specialist will usually take note of the referrals designated as urgent by the family doctor. Obviously a family doctor who abuses this facility will find that after a while even his 'urgent' referrals may be waiting long periods.

Home visits

There is one other way in which a general practitioner can obtain an urgent consultation for a patient with a specialist and that is to ask for what is called a home or domiciliary visit. Specialists rather tend to like making domiciliary visits because they are entitled to claim an additional fee from the government. This service is expensive in terms of specialists' time but convenient for the patient. Domiciliary visits are sometimes requested where patients cannot leave their own homes without a considerable amount of upheaval, and they may be requested by a GP who wants a specialist to assist him in his treatment of a particular condition.

When things go wrong

The referral system between GPs and consultant specialists sometimes leads to misunderstandings between family doctors and their patients.

The major cause of dissent usually results from a doctor's failure or reluctance to arrange a referral. Theoretically it is the GP's responsibility to decide when a specialist opinion is required. Some practitioners guard their right to refer jealously and will not refer unless they are genuinely in desperate need of advice or help. Others are less rigid and will happily refer patients who may feel that a second opinion is desirable for one reason or another.

Since a patient will only actively request a second opinion on a medical problem if he is dissatisfied in some way with the treatment or advice he has been given by his own family doctor,

The top ten referrals most commonly made by GPs

1 Hospital out-patient departments

2 Laboratories, for basic blood or urine tests

3 Radiological departments, for chest X-rays

4 Laboratories, for more complex tests

5 Radiology departments, for ordinary X-rays apart from chest X-rays

6 Radiology departments, for contrast media X-rays such as barium meals (see p. 186)

7 Direct hospital admissions

8 Health visitors, social service departments, etc.

9 Private consultations

10 Hospital casualty departments

The top ten consultants most commonly used by GPs

1 General surgeons

2 General physicians

3 Obstetricians

4 Gynaecologists

5 Orthopaedic surgeons

6 Ear, nose and throat specialists

7 Paediatricians

8 Psychiatrists

9 Geriatricians

10 Ophthalmic surgeons

sensitive practitioners regard such a request as something of a calculated insult. It seems to me that this is unreasonable and that any patient who asks for a second opinion should be entitled to have one. Requests for referrals to surgeons specializing in cosmetic operations should always be met since without a referral letter a patient may be tempted to visit a surgeon who may not be properly qualified.

Another cause of confusion is the fact that patients often assume that the specialist is in some way superior to the GP. The truth is that a GP does not hand over responsibility for his patient to the specialist when he arranges a referral; he merely asks for technical support. A capable GP will on occasions disagree with the treatment programme outlined by specialists. It is an important duty of the family doctor to act as an interpreter for the patient, explaining procedures which may have been advocated and discussing the advantages and disadvantages of proposed forms of treatment. He should understand the individual patient's circumstances, capabilities and needs better than anyone else and should be in a position to provide the patient with an expert outside opinion as a 'friend' of the family. Good family doctors are not always well liked by their specialist colleagues in the hospital service.

Variations

A final point worth making about general practitioner referrals is that there are enormous differences between the referral rates of different family doctors. One survey showed that whereas one practitioner referred patients to specialist psychiatrists at the rate of 17 patients per 10,000, patients seen by another had a referral rate of 160 per 10,000.

These variations do not necessarily mean that there were more psychiatric problems in the second doctor's practice, nor do they tell us anything about the general capabilities of the doctors concerned. A high referral rate does not necessarily show that a general practitioner is a good or a bad doctor. For example, a GP who is particularly interested in psychological problems but not particularly interested in gynaecology may see most of his psychiatric problems himself but have a high referral rate to local gynaecologists. Such variations merely exhibit good sense on the GP's part. After all, the single most important criterion in general practice is that the family doctor should know when he does not know, and should recognize his own capabilities and his own limitations.

The primary care team

Gone are the days when the general practitioner worked alone. Today the list of people working with him makes a football team coach look a positive loner. There are nurses, bath attendants, receptionists, social workers, health visitors, telephonists and representatives of an apparently endless series of supplementary professions. Some of them do work which helps the patient, some of them do work which helps the doctor and some of them do work which does not seem to be of any real value to anyone other than themselves.

The various members of the primary care team can be put into two categories. In the first group are those workers who have administrative duties and no clinical responsibilities at all. In the second are those whose duties are mainly clinical.

Receptionists

A decade or two ago general practitioners used to manage all their administrative chores themselves. Today the GP who tried to manage without any administrative help would be quite unable to provide his patients with anything approaching the quality of clinical care patients are entitled to expect. The number of forms in use in the health service has reached extraordinary proportions and simply sorting and filing the morning mail is a time-consuming task. In addition to dealing with the mail, doctors' receptionists are usually expected to be able to take telephone calls, pass on messages, sort patients' notes out of the files, look after the appointments book, deal with requests for repeat prescriptions and carry out the other hundred and one essential but non-clinical chores involved in an ordinary general practice.

Occasionally doctors' receptionists have nursing qualifications, but most do not, and should not be tempted or expected to offer clinical advice or make decisions dependent upon clinical knowledge.

Doctors are expected to hire and pay for their own reception staff but a large proportion of the cost of such assistance can be reclaimed from the government.

Since general practitioners are bound under the terms of their contracts to provide cover for their patients 24 hours a day, and since it is not easy to find staff willing to answer telephones during the night, most general practitioners arrange for their telephone calls to be put through to their own homes outside surgery hours. This is done in various ways: sometimes the telephone switchboard operator is instructed to intercept calls; sometimes a switching device is used to divert calls automatically from the surgery number to a private number; and sometimes a telephone answering machine is employed to give an alternative number.

Secretaries and practice managers

In view of the large number of letters which have to be written and the fact that most general practitioners have well-nigh illegible handwriting, most practices employ a typist or secretary. The responsibilities of the secretary can vary enormously from very simple and straightforward chores to dealing with just about every administrative detail involved in the practice. Larger practices where there are several partners and where there may be a dozen or more receptionists (most of them working part-time) may employ a practice manager who will have total administrative control of the staff, the building maintenance and all the administration of the practice, including the hiring of locum doctors, the requisition of official and private stationery and the management of the practice finances. Since a three- or four-man practice may deal with over 20,000 surgery consultations in a year, and since the total amount of money passing through the partnership may approach £100,000, the responsibilities of a practice manager are clearly considerable.

District nurses

The doctor's most important clinical partner is naturally the nurse. In each community area there will be a number of publicly employed nurses who may be known either as district nurses or home nurses. Some district nurses are state registered (SRNs) while others are state enrolled (SENs). The first of these two qualifications is considered academically superior to the second, and nurses who are registered as opposed to enrolled are usually entitled to perform a small number of additional duties denied to the enrolled nurse.

It is impossible to prepare a comprehensive list of the duties of a district nurse since the duties obviously vary from area to area, practice to practice, and nurse to nurse, but both grades of nurse are usually considered qualified to give injections, change dressings, give douches and enemas, take swabs and syringe ears. Usually only registered nurses are allowed to take blood samples. Catheterizations and checking blood pressures are additional duties often performed by district nurses. Unhappily statistics show that many district nurses spend more time travelling than they do with their patients, and even when they get to their patients they spend a considerable amount of time on mundane chores such as giving bed baths, cutting nails, and supervising bathing in the bathroom. Whether these are duties which truly need the skills of a trained nurse is doubtful. In some areas specialist bath attendants are employed.

Practice nurses

Today many general practitioners employ their own practice nurses who work with them in their surgeries. As with other ancilliary staff members the doctor can claim back part of the nurse's salary from the government. Surgery nurses' duties are generally similar to those of the district nurse (giving injections, taking blood samples, syringing ears, checking blood pressures, changing dressings, taking swabs, and so on) but in addition they may occasionally be expected to chaperone a doctor contemplating an intimate examination of an unusually delicate or imaginative patient.

Midwives and health visitors

There are two other types of qualified nurse involved in primary care. The midwife's role is, I suppose, obvious enough. It is her task to look after pregnant women, to attend them during labour and delivery and to provide the new mother and her baby with immediate medical care. In practice the way in which the midwife provides care varies according to a number of different factors. Most important of these factors is the attitude of the general practitioner with whom the midwife works. If the GP prefers to have his pregnant patients delivered at home then the midwife will have a high proportion of home confinements to look after. If the GP provides only ante-natal care and hands over all deliveries to the local maternity hospital then she may well attend very few deliveries. If the GP refers some patients to hospital obstetricians but allows other patients to have babies in hospital under his care (and this only happens in areas where GPs are allowed access to maternity wards) the midwife will attend deliveries often enough but may attend few in the home.

The function of the health visitor is far less clearly defined than that of the midwife. It is claimed that health visitors spend their time counselling young mothers before and after childbirth but at least one recent survey showed that health visitors spend more than half their time on administration, travelling, training and eating.

In some areas there are also domiciliary physio- and occupational therapists who can be asked to visit patients at home and assist in rehabilitation e.g. after a stroke, chest illness or accident.

Home helps

Of the numerous employees who are provided by the local authority (through its social services department) the most important are undoubtedly the home helps who, by performing simple but often arduous chores, enable the elderly to remain independent and at home.

The average GP

Statistics about general practitioners abound. The medical libraries are stuffed to the ceilings with books and journals analysing the activities of GPs and the habits of patients. The only thing that all these surveys show is that there is just as much variety among GPs as you might expect and that your chances of finding 'the average GP' are about as good as those of the GP finding 'the average patient'.

The purpose of this section is simply to give patients a brief introduction to general practice and to help both patients and doctors get some idea of what to expect from an 'average sort of general practitioner'.

To begin with, the accumulated figures show that although only 15 per cent of family doctors now work in single-handed practice less than 50 per cent work in groups of more than three. Seventy-five per cent of all practices have appointment systems, and most town and city practices employ deputizing services for at least some of the emergency duty time. A quarter of all family doctors have hospital jobs and a third of all practices employ their own nurses.

Most general practitioners have between 2000 and 2500 patients to look after and the 'average' patient will be seen three times a year in the surgery and once every two years at home. In an average sort of year the average sort of doctor with an average list of patients will see 1000 patients in their own homes and about 6000 patients in his surgery. Since some patients do not get seen at all for years at a time it is no surprise to discover that in a 12-month period a doctor will not see a third of his patients at all. And 13 per cent of the entire list of patients will take up more than half his working time.

The average general practitioner will practise in a converted house which he shares with his two partners (see p. 40). He will take four weeks' holiday a year and be on duty for two nights a week and for one weekend a month. He will spend 20 hours a week in his surgery seeing patients; 10 hours a week visiting patients who have requested daytime visits; 10 hours a week writing and answering letters and dealing with other aspects of practice administration. He will therefore work a basic 40-hour week but on top of that he will be on call for an average of about 48 hours, giving a working week of 88 hours. (Being on call is more exhausting than may be generally thought. Even if there are few calls the doctor must remain alert – like a runner permanently stuck on the starting blocks. Firemen and policemen will confirm that in these circumstances a little action is sometimes a relief.)

The average doctor's working day

Morning surgery

A total of twenty patients to be seen:

1 Woman wanting a repeat prescription for her contraceptive pill.
2 Mother with two small children both of whom are alleged to have worms.
3 Elderly man with a cough that has been present for six days.
4 Boy of twelve years who has been bitten by a dog.
5 Elderly lady needing blood pressure check and repeat of her prescription.
6 Woman of thirty-five who bursts into tears as soon as she enters the surgery and who is clearly suffering from depression.
7 Man of forty who complains of backache.

8 Woman of fifty with slight chest symptoms.

9 Girl of nineteen with sore throat.

10 Mother with small boy aged five who has earache and a skin rash.

11 Mother with two-month-old baby with feeding problem.

12 Eighty-year-old man complaining of deafness.

13 Twenty-eight-year-old man complaining of persistent headaches.

14 Woman of thirty-five who cannot sleep.

15 Woman of fifty-five who has pains in her left knee and feels tired.

16 Man of twenty-six wanting Heavy Goods Vehicle Licence Examination.

17 Woman of twenty-nine with cold symptoms, mild skin rash, painful periods, bad breath, piles and a small varicose vein.

18 Man requiring sick note for a period six weeks ago.

19 Mother with small boy who has been complaining of abdominal pain for two days.

20 Man complaining of intermittent chest pains present for a week.

During the surgery there may be eight telephone calls to be answered:

1 Woman wanting a home visit for her husband who has had chest trouble for three days.

2 Woman awaiting the result of a pregnancy test.

3 Woman whose child has earache.

4 Man whose wife has been ill in bed with stomach pains for two days.

5 Social worker wanting information about the parents of a baby admitted to hospital.

6 Woman wanting a sick note to cover her husband who has been off work after an operation.

7 Woman wanting to know whether she can get pregnant if she is two hours late taking her contraceptive pill.

8 Woman wondering why the hospital hasn't sent her husband an appointment for his prostate gland operation.

Immediately after the surgery there may be fourteen repeat prescriptions to sign, four letters to write and a miscellaneous bundle of hospital letters and pathology laboratory result forms to study.

Then there will be the home visits

1   The man who has had chest trouble for three days.
2   The woman whose child has earache.
3   The woman who has been ill in bed with stomach pains for two days.
4   An elderly lady whose blood pressure needs checking.

Evening surgery

A total of eighteen patients to be seen:

1   Man wanting a sick note for three days off work with a cold.
2   Boy with a sore throat brought by his mother who wants a prescription for her contraceptive pill.
3   Man with aches and pains in his shoulders and back.
4   Woman of forty who has been constipated for a week.
5   Woman of thirty-four with a lump in her left breast.
6   Man of twenty-six with pains which he thinks are due to indigestion.
7   Man of fifty-seven requiring a blood pressure check and some cough medicine.
8   Man of twenty-two with acne spots.
9   Woman of seventeen wanting to go on the contraceptive pill.
10   Woman of eighty-four who wants her ears syringing.
11   Man of fifty wanting to know the results of X-rays of his chest.
12   Woman of twenty-six who thinks she may be pregnant.
13   Mother with small small children both of whom have colds and coughs.
14   Mother with daughter who has catarrh.
15   Man of thirty-eight who has been suffering from diarrhoea for four days.

16 Woman of forty-five who complains of feeling tired all the time.
17 Woman of twenty-three who has earache and a vaginal infection.
18 Woman of sixty-four requiring blood pressure check and a prescription for her pills.

During this surgery there may be five telephone calls:

1 Woman of twenty-two awaiting result of urine test.
2 Mother with child who has had a temperature for two days.
3 Mother with child who has had abdominal pain for one day.
4 Man of sixty-six wanting to know if he can have a prescription for a bottle of cough medicine.
5 Woman of thirty-eight wondering why she has not heard from the hospital about her gall bladder operation.

There will as usual have been a number of calls requiring appointments, repeat prescriptions and so on which will all have been dealt with by the receptionists.

The woman with the child who has abdominal pains may agree to bring the child in to surgery to be seen at the end of the formal list of patients. The woman with the child who has had a temperature will be visited at home after the end of the surgery.

Of course if each problem was as neatly defined as it has been here the work would be ridiculously easy. Unfortunately life is not always what it seems and a minor symptom may hide some more serious illness. For example, the man who attended the morning surgery with a cough that had been present for six days may have been coughing up blood. He may also have lost a considerable amount of weight and admit, after further questioning, that his cough had in fact been present for more like three months. The woman with slight chest symptoms may really have come for advice about her younger son who has been getting into trouble with the police quite frequently. She may be depressed about this and about the fact that her husband is still drinking far too much. The mother with the two-month-old baby with a feeding problem may still not have had a period and may suspect that she is pregnant again. The woman of fifty-three who has pains in her left knee and feels tired may admit to having been suicidally depressed for two weeks. At the evening surgery the woman who wants her contraceptive pills may turn out to have developed a varicose vein in her left leg. She may be cross when the doctor refuses to provide a prescription for the pills. The woman of forty who has been constipated for a week may eventually admit that she has also passed a little blood and reluctantly agree to be examined. The woman of twenty-six who thinks she may be pregnant may insist that she will want an abortion is she is. And at least a third of the patients seen will have psychological problems in addition to their purely physical symptoms. And if the day is a little more hectic than average there may well be an emergency call during the morning surgery. The doctor may have to abandon his patients to visit a known diabetic who has collapsed in her own living room. When that has been dealt with the other patients will still have to be seen.

The average doctor's annual workload

In an average sort of year an average sort of doctor with an average sort of list (i.e. about 2500 patients) will deal with the following problems:

500 coughs, colds and upper respiratory tract infections	50 bad backs
	40 pregnancies
	30 cases of migraine
300 emotional upsets	26 deaths
250 attacks of diarrhoea	25 cases of hay fever
200 skin problems	25 high blood pressure cases
100 bouts of tonsillitis	
100 attacks of rheumatism	7 heart attacks
75 ear infections	5 acute appendicitis cases
50 attacks of cystitis	5 strokes
50 bouts of bronchitis	5 newly diagnosed cancers

Getting to see the doctor

Patients who are old enough to remember the good old days before the beginning of the National Health Service claim that seeing the doctor never used to be a problem. If you were fit enough you dragged yourself along to the surgery where you sat in the waiting room until your turn came. If you were too ill to go out then you stayed at home and sent a message for the doctor to visit you. It was all delightfully simple.

The introduction of modern administrative aids, auxilliary workers and vocational training has been accompanied by a number of changes in the way in which doctors and patients meet. Many patients feel that the changes have been for the worse.

Home visiting

I will begin with the question of home visiting which is a perennial cause of discontent among patients. It is an indisputable fact that the number of home visits made by general practitioners has fallen quite considerably in recent years and still seems to be falling consistently.

GPs argue that this trend is justifiable since the majority of patients wanting to be seen at home are physically able to visit the surgery. Small children, for example, can be safely transported from home to surgery even when suffering from throat and ear infections. The advantages, claim the doctors, are that the patient will be seen in the building where the equipment is and that the GP will have more time to spend on each patient. It is certainly a fact that a doctor can see four or five patients in a surgery in the time it takes to visit one patient at home.

The routine visiting of patients, claim those who would prefer to see most of their patients in the surgery building, should be done by other less highly qualified people. Home visiting, they say, is a leftover from the days when GPs used to perform surgical operations on the kitchen table.

Patients and doctors who oppose this trend do so on various grounds. It is sometimes claimed that by seeing the patient in his home environment the GP can learn a great deal more about the patient's physical and mental state. It is argued that old people benefit because if the GP does not visit them no one else will. And it is argued that it is the doctor's responsibility and duty to see the patient wherever he wants to be seen.

There are, of course, no clear answers to this argument and there will undoubtedly be disagreement for some time to come about the rights and wrongs of home visiting. The main danger, I suspect, is that at some time in the future doctors will stop doing home visits altogether. After all, Britain is one of the few countries in the world where doctors do still see patients in their homes. This would in my view be tragic since emergency home visiting is an extremely important facet of general practice, and the treatment of ill and convalescent patients at home will undoubtedly become more and more important in future years as the shortage of hospital beds becomes more apparent.

Meanwhile, the disputes about home visiting would probably be less emotive if patients would remember that visits should only be requested when invalids are in need of medical attention and cannot attend the surgery because of illness. I suspect that a number of the patients who complain about doctors refusing to visit have been under the misapprehension that it is the doctor's duty to call, even if the patient is fit enough to attend the surgery but considers that a home visit would be more convenient for social reasons. Doctors, on the other hand, have to remember that visits are sometimes requested unnecessarily because patients misinterpret physical signs.

Visits to the surgery

Getting seen in the doctor's surgery is another problem which many patients seem to find worrying. When appointment systems were introduced into general medical practice about thirty years ago it was immediately clear that there would be advantages and disadvantages for both doctors and patients.

Many patients complained that the old style 'free for all' surgeries had led to enormous waiting times and had contributed to the exchange of infectious diseases. Initially, at any rate, they welcomed appointment systems as a way of avoiding both these problems.

Doctors welcomed the idea of appointment systems (and introduced them into their practices at a rapid rate during the 1950s and 60s) because they felt that seeing patients by appointment would enable them to regulate their professional life far more efficiently. Introducing appointment systems into general practice meant that new waiting rooms did not have to be as large, that the work could be spread throughout the week, and that holidays could be organized with less trouble. Doctors also realized that by giving their patients appointments they could arrange to see patients with specific problems in particular surgery sessions and that by being able to allot appointment times to patients they could allow longer periods of time for individuals with difficult problems.

Unfortunately, no one had realized that there were various reasons why appointment systems should not work as well in general practice as they do in other walks of life. The most important point, of course, is that a large proportion of the people needing to see a GP need to see him urgently. Dentists, accountants and lawyers have few urgent problems to deal with. Doctors in general practice regularly see problems considered to be urgent by those who are suffering.

Whereas a client ringing up a solicitor to make an appointment would be very satisfied if given an appointment one week ahead, a patient ringing up a doctor is likely to consider it a disaster if offered an appointment so far in the future. And a disaster it may well be, of course.

This simple difficulty is just one of the problems. It is also a fact of life that patients visiting GPs need very different amounts of time spent on them. One patient needs two minutes and another patient needs an hour. In addition there is the risk that before or during a surgery session a doctor may be called out to make an urgent home visit. When this happens the appointments are effectively valueless. All these individual problems are compounded by the fact that, justifiably or not, the workload on GPs is such that appointments are usually booked at intervals of five minutes. A consultation that takes twenty minutes can create havoc.

Patients seem on the whole to find the appointments system in many surgeries a disaster. They complain that it may take a week to get an appointment, that a visit to the surgery now involves either two visits or a visit and a telephone call, and that the receptionists have too much responsibility when it comes to handing out urgent appointments.

I suspect that these complaints are often justified. Sometimes, however, I suspect that they are not. For example, I think it is unfair for a patient demanding an urgent appointment to expect to see a particular doctor at a particular time. I believe that every patient requesting an urgent appointment should be guaranteed an appointment on the same day but I do not see how any system can be organized which would guarantee a convenient appointment with a specific doctor.

Doctors probably have to reconcile themselves to the fact that as long as appointment systems exist they are bound to annoy some of the people some of the time. For example, the accessible doctor who agrees to see every patient who wants to be seen will often need to work more quickly than he would like, and may frequently find that his system has broken down, with the result that patients complain that despite having made appointments they must still sit in the waiting room for three-quarters of an hour. On the other hand, the inaccessible doctor who insists on seeing a fixed number of patients at regular intervals will undoubtedly annoy those patients who cannot be seen for six days. The doctor who works his five-minute appointment system effectively may miss the odd serious depression or incipient heart attack while the doctor who spends forty minutes on a five-minute patient will probably raise the blood pressure of those still waiting.

The top ten reasons for going to see a GP

1 Respiratory tract symptoms, e.g. coughs, colds and sore throats

2 Nervous system disorders, mental symptoms and emotional problems

3 Problems with the circulatory system, e.g. blood pressure, bad circulation and chest pains

4 Digestive system problems, e.g. indigestion, constipation and diarrhoea

5 Skin problems, e.g. rashes, spots and ulcers

6 Rheumatic conditions, e.g. joint and muscle pains and backaches

7 Accidents, e.g. cuts, dog bites and broken bones

8 'Something not quite right': generally ill-defined condition which remains a mystery after consultation

9 To get a sick note

10 Genito-urinary system disorders, e.g. cystitis, bladder troubles and kidney problems

Telephone consultations

There is a third way in which patients can get in touch with their doctors – by telephone – and I suspect that this method has not yet been properly utilized.

Some family doctors refuse to take telephone calls at all. Some refuse to take telephone calls during surgery hours. Some take telephone calls at any time. There are arguments in favour of both the second and third of these alternatives. A nice compromise is for the doctor to agree to take calls at any time but always to insist on completing a consultation in progress before talking to a telephone caller. Many consultations which do not require physical examinations can be conducted safely, effectively, and to the satisfaction of both doctor and patient with the aid of the telephone.

Getting to see the doctor: points to remember

1 A home visit should be requested before 10.00 a.m., and should be requested because the patient is physically unable to attend the surgery and not because a home visit is more convenient.

2 When making urgent or emergency calls it is important to make the urgency clear to the receptionist and to give the full address.

3 A patient who needs what he considers to be an urgent consultation is entitled to be seen within 24 hours. It is not a receptionist's job to decide whether a consultation is urgent.

4 When an urgent appointment has been requested it is probably unrealistic to expect to be given an appointment at a given time with a specific doctor.

5 When booking routine appointments it is important to book for each member of a family to be seen, and, where medical examinations (e.g. for life insurance purposes) are required, this should be stated when the appointment is booked.

The consultation

Judging from the number of patients I see who pause, just as they are about to disappear through the door, and ask me 'just one final question' or tell me a late remembered symptom, there must be many patients who leave their general practitioner's surgery and metaphorically kick themselves when they remember a point they forgot to make or a question they forgot to ask.

Whether we recognize it or not a visit to the doctor is for many people a rather frightening event. And with consultations rarely lasting more than five minutes or so it is easy for a vital question or important piece of information to be overlooked.

So it is always wise to spend a few moments thinking about what you want to tell the doctor – and what you expect from the doctor in return. Do not be frightened or embarrassed to make notes beforehand and to add to them during the consultation. Doctors write down the information that you give them – there is no reason why you shouldn't jot down what you get in return.

I have prepared two check lists to help.

What to tell the doctor

1 All the symptoms that you have noticed, even if they do not seem relevant to you. Your doctor does not expect you to be able to differentiate between the relevant and the irrelevant. That is his job. And sometimes an apparently stray clue may lead to a diagnosis.

2 When the symptoms first started. If the symptoms have recurred several times it helps if you can tell the doctor the dates. Women with gynaecological problems or obstetric problems should be prepared to provide information about the dates of their last period.

3 Details of any remedies you have tried, and whether or not they had any effect.

4 Any family history that you think might be relevant. If there is a family history of diabetes, for example, it is important to tell the doctor. Even if you think that he already knows it does not do any harm to remind him.

5 If you have not seen the doctor before and he might not have had a chance to look through your notes you should tell him about any past medical events which might be relevant. A man with chest pains, for example, should mention it if he has had an operation for a peptic ulcer. A woman with abdominal pains should say if she has had a hysterectomy.

6 About any recent trips abroad. Diseases not normally seen in your own country can be brought back from even the briefest trip.

What to ask the doctor

1 What he thinks is wrong with you. It's your body and your illness and there is nothing wrong in asking the doctor what he thinks is wrong. However, if you ask you must be prepared for the answer. And remember that at the end of a large proportion of consultations your GP will not have made a firm diagnosis. So do not be disappointed if he tells you that he does not know.

2 Whether you need to see him again, and if so when.

3 If any tests are to be arranged or any hospital appointments made, whether you have to make arrangements yourself.

4 As much as you can about the treatment that is recommended. If pills or medicine of any kind are prescribed then you should find out how often the medicine is to be taken, whether it has to be taken before or after meals, whether the whole course has to be completed and whether there are special side effects of which you should be aware (see p. 210).

5 Whether any other advice needs to be followed – if a special diet is required, for example.

Ten ways to keep your doctor sane

1 Do not phone at 5.00 a.m. to say that you have mild cystitis that has been troubling you for a week

2 Do not refuse to take the pills that have been prescribed and then complain that you are no better

3 Do not tell him that you have just read about a wonderful new drug in your daily newspaper and you would like his opinion of it

4 Do not take the children with you when you have booked a single appointment and, when he has finished dealing with the last of them, ask if he has Aunt Thelma's blood test results

5 Do not wear six layers of clothes when you visit the surgery with a chest complaint or try to undo the buttons without taking your gloves off

6 Do not telephone at 9.30 on a Sunday evening to ask for a repeat prescription

7 Do not stop him in the street and ask him when you are going to hear from the hospital

8 Do not insist that you pay your national insurance stamps and are entitled to any treatment you want

9 Do not point out that you have a friend who has a friend on the Regional Health Authority medical committee and so you think you are entitled to be treated as a private patient

10 Do not insist on a home visit and then go out shopping and, when you get back and find his irate note, ring the surgery and demand another visit

Forms and certificates used by the GP

The majority of contacts between patients and GPs result in the exchange of one or more pieces of paper. The total number of forms which can be found in or on a GP's desk is extremely high but the following forms and certificates are the ones most commonly used in general practice.

Form FP10
The ordinary prescription form.

Form FP95
Can be obtained from Post Offices. Patients who need to visit the doctor regularly but who are not entitled to exemption from prescription fees should obtain this form and buy a 'pre-payment certificate' or NHS season ticket.

Form FP91
If you think you may be exempt from prescription charges ask at a Post Office for this form (see p. 204).

Form M11
If you suspect that you may be exempt from prescription charges because your income is low ask for this form at a Post Office (see p. 204).

Form FP4
This is the official name given to an ordinary NHS medical card. In theory a patient who visits a GP without a Form FP4 can be charged a fee which the patient can then claim back from the Family Practitioner Committee. The GP must give an official receipt when taking the fee. In practice I doubt if this happens very often however.

Form FP1
A patient who wishes to register with a doctor but has lost his medical card can register with the aid of this form, which will be supplied by the GP.

Form FP58
This small pink card is the one used to register a newborn baby with a GP. If the FP58 has been lost an ordinary FP1 can be used instead.

Form FP13
Anyone leaving the army, navy or air force will be given a copy of this form to hand to his or her new GP.

Form FP19
If you need to see a doctor away from home the doctor will probably ask you to complete this form. He will then write your clinical details on the back of the form, which will be used to ensure that he receives payment from the NHS for treating you and to inform your own GP of the treatment provided. In holiday resort areas many GPs obtain a large proportion of their income in this way.

Form FP32
Should you need to ask a GP other than the one with whom you are registered for emergency treatment you may be required to help him complete this form, which will entitle him to claim a fee.

Form Med 3
A social security sick note. There is no fee payable for the provision of this sick note, which is intended for use by the social security office only.

Form Med 5
If a sick note was not issued when a patient was ill, this form can be used to provide retrospective cover. It can also be used when the doctor has not himself seen the patient (for example, when a patient has just been discharged from hospital).

Form Med A (in Scotland Form 11)
If a GP feels able to provide a death
certificate this is the form he will use.
There is no fee for its provision.

Form Mat B1
After the 26th week of pregnancy an
expectant mother may receive one of
these forms, also known as a
certificate of expected confinement
(see p. 313).

Form Mat B2
After delivery a young mother may be
given one of these forms known as
certificates of confinement (see
p. 313).

Form FW8
Any woman whose pregnancy has
been confirmed is entitled to a copy
of this form, which is effectively a
prescription charge exemption
certificate but which also entitles the
expectant mother to free dental
treatment and free milk.

Form FP1001 (in Scotland EC102)
A woman who wants her GP to
provide her with contraceptive advice
or treatment will be asked to complete
a copy of this form, which enables the
GP to claim a special fee.

Form FP1003 (in Scotland EC104)
A woman who wants contraceptive
advice (as opposed to ordinary
medical treatment) while away from
home will be asked to complete one
of these forms.

Form DP32
An application form to register as a
disabled person. A doctor may charge
a fee for this form, which the patient
must pay.

Form FP81 (in Northern Ireland
NV/1)
When a doctor visits a patient between
the hours of 11.00 p.m. and 7.00 a.m.
he is entitled to claim a night visit fee.
The patient must, however, sign the
form to confirm that the doctor has
visited.

The list above does not include the forms used for referring patients to hospitals (for
an opinion, an X-ray or a laboratory test), since these forms vary from area to area.
Nor does it include the enormous variety of other forms commonly presented to GPs
for completion, either by patients or on their behalf. Some of these 'unofficial' forms
are described below:

Private sick note
Can be written on any piece of headed
notepaper or specially printed form.
There will be a fee payable by the
patient.

**Immunization or vaccination
certificate**
Official International Certificates of
Vaccination against cholera are
obtainable but a fee has to be paid.
(The vaccination itself is provided free
when it is required on medical

grounds, e.g. the traveller is going to a
country where cholera is endemic.)
Fees are also charged for signing
other vaccination certificates such as
those produced by airlines.

Employment medical report
The employer will usually provide the
form and will often (but not always)
pay the doctor's fee. The fee may be
lower if the employee is paying since
many doctors like to see themselves as
modern-day Robin Hoods.

Emigration medical report
Forms vary from country to country
and the fee usually has to be paid by
the person wishing to emigrate.

Life insurance medical report
Doctors are sometimes asked to
complete 'short reports' on their
patients for life insurance companies.
(Most insurance company application
forms include a clause which
automatically gives the company the
right to obtain this information.) When
a medical examination is required a
longer form will have to be completed.
The companies usually pay for both
long and short reports.

**Sickness or accident insurance
claim form**
The form is usually provided by the
insurance company but the doctor's
fee is usually the responsibility of the
patient.

**Elderly driver's medical
examination certificate**
Some insurance companies expect
elderly drivers to have medical
examinations. The doctor's fee usually
has to be paid by the patient.

Disabled driver's certificate
Forms are provided by the local social
services department, who should pay
any fee involved. When completed,
this certificate entitles the driver to an
orange badge, the value of which
varies from area to area.

**Public service vehicle and heavy
goods vehicle medical certificates**
Before being allowed to drive a bus or
lorry an individual must have a medical

examination. The fee may be paid by
the employer but is usually the
responsibility of the driver.

**Racing driver's medical
certificate**
The fee is usually the responsibility of
the driver.

Report for a solicitor
With a patient's permission a GP will
write a report for a solicitor. The
solicitor will pay the fee but the
patient will naturally pay the solicitor
in the end.

Exemption from jury service
A court form will be completed and
there is not usually any fee.

Passport form application
GPs are often asked to sign these
forms as referees. Photographs also
have to be verified and the patient
must have known the GP for at least
two years. A fee is usually payable by
the patient.

Adoption medical reports
These vary from area to area and from
agency to agency. Prospective
parents are sometimes expected
to pay the fees.

Police reports
Doctors are sometimes asked to
complete and sign forms for individuals
accused of driving while under the
influence of alcohol. They may also
sign forms required by individuals
applying for shotgun certificates.

There are many other statutory and non-statutory forms available which require the
attention of a GP. A fully comprehensive list would take up a disproportionate amount
of space since most of the forms and certificates are self-explanatory. The forms
GPs use to apply for payment or to report sickness to any of the official agencies are
available through the local Family Practitioner Committee.

Choosing your doctor

Qualified, registered medical practitioners (whether they are in private practice or working within the health service) are not allowed to advertise. This means not only that they cannot promote themselves on billboards or television, but that they are not allowed to provide potential patients with any more than the most rudimentary details about their qualifications, experience and interest. I do not know what value this restriction on advertising has, but there is of course one enormous disadvantage for patients, in that there is no single easy way for them to differentiate between various practitioners in the same area.

Professional status

The first and by far the most important thing for a patient to look for when contemplating joining a doctor's list is proof of his professional status. It is illegal for anyone who does not have acceptable medical qualifications to claim to be a registered medical practitioner and, in addition, it is illegal for any registered medical practitioner who has not obtained an official certificate confirming that he has completed the appropriate period of training to practise as a principal in an NHS general practice. Local Family Practitioner Committees publish lists of practitioners who satisfy these criteria, and copies of these lists can be seen in General Post Offices. Local telephone directories also usually carry lists of general practitioners under the heading 'Physicians and Surgeons'.

There are no local or national bodies from whom lists of private general practitioners can be obtained but all registered medical practitioners, whether in NHS or private practice, will be listed on the Medical Register and in the Medical Directory, one or both of which can be found in the reference sections of most local libraries. From 1982 the Medical Directory will identify GPs taking private patients.

Official directories usually (but not invariably) contain details of the qualifications of practitioners. All general medical practitioners must have the basic qualifications, but a growing number have specialist qualifications as well. Details of which groups of letters mean what can be found at the back of this book on pp. 334 ff. Unfortunately for the patient seeking a suitable practitioner, these qualifications are of little practical value since a doctor who also happens to be a qualified surgeon is not necessarily a good or even competent general practitioner. Some doctors may have many diplomas but remain professionally inadequate.

The qualification considered by some to be most relevant to general practice is membership of the Royal College of General Practitioners. Founded comparatively recently, in 1953, the College has taken upon itself the task of turning general practice into a recognized medical speciality. Originally, practising family doctors were allowed to join the College without taking any examination, but today potential members must pass a series of tests. Any doctor who has been a member of the Royal College of General Practitioners for five years, and who can persuade three colleagues who are already fellows of the College to propose him, can apply for fellowship.

Technical competence

Most patients would obviously like to select a practitioner who is technically competent. Unfortunately, once again, it is difficult to suggest any way in which competence can be judged.

The Medical Directory may list the research papers that a doctor has published, but publications mean nothing at all in the context of daily practice. Local consultant specialists and junior hospital doctors could probably provide you with much biased information, but their criteria for judging a general practitioner are not necessarily those which might be adopted by a would-be patient. For one thing, the patient needs a general practitioner with a wide range of skills, whereas the specialist sees only one aspect of the general practitioner's work. And, for another thing, the good specialist and the good general practitioner will not necessarily share the same aims as far as their

patients are concerned. Good general practitioners must sometimes make enemies of hospital practitioners. (I am not suggest-
ing that family doctors and hospital specialists must inevitably
be at each other's throats, but that they will occasionally fail to
agree simply because their views of what may be best for any
one patient must occasionally vary.)

Seeking advice and information from friends and neighbours
who may have already experienced the services provided by
local GPs is a more reliable way to form an opinion, but there
will undoubtedly be many conflicting views. Some patients will
have nothing but praise, others will be critical. By talking to a
number of people, however, it should be possible to acquire
some sort of reliable impression and decide whether the practitioner you are considering offers impersonal efficiency, friendly
chaos, or an acceptable mixture of both. In addition you should
be able to find out a little about the special skills or interests of
local doctors.

How the practice is run

There are, of course, many differences in the ways in which
individual practices are organized, and a few telephone calls
should provide the patient looking for a doctor with information
about the ways in which separate practices are administered:
whether, for example, appointment systems are used or not.
Some patients may find the presence or absence of an appointment system enough to make a practice desirable but the truth,
I'm afraid, is that the vast variety of statistics which exist in
medical libraries show that there is absolutely no relationship
between the way in which a practice is structured and the quality
or effectiveness of the care provided.

Where the surgery is

The geographical location of a doctor's surgery is an obvious
factor to be taken into consideration. In some urban areas there
may be half a dozen separate practice premises within range but

in many rural areas there will be but one surgery available. There is little point in electing to become a patient on the list of a wonderful doctor if you have to make a four-hour bus journey every time you need advice.

Other considerations

The sex, age or nationality of a potential doctor may be of paramount importance and, for example, the patient who will be happy only with a female doctor or a Hindu doctor may find that his choice of practitioner is strictly limited. Such self-imposed limitations obviously make choosing a new doctor a relatively simple process.

Changing your doctor

It is an important right of both doctors and patients to be able to choose the individuals with whom they have a professional relationship. Trust, faith and respect are vital qualities for any doctor-patient relationship, and where these qualities are lacking it is better for all concerned if the relationship is terminated. The simple, unavoidable, indisputable truth is that no single individual can possibly have qualities which satisfy or attract all other individuals. One patient's ideal doctor may be another patient's idea of a one-man disaster area.

In theory, at least, it is relatively simple for a patient to change doctors. In practice, I recognize that there can often be problems. I will deal first with the basic facts.

Registering with a new doctor

To register with a doctor in general practice who has his own list of patients, an individual must simply present himself with his medical card (known as an FP4 – see p. 67) at the doctor's surgery. Indeed the patient does not have to see the doctor at all but can simply leave his card at the surgery. The patient who has lost his medical card can register by obtaining a card called an FP1, either from the local Family Practitioner Committee or from the doctor whose list he intends to join. Naturally no patient can be on the list of more than one doctor at a time and joining one doctor's list usually means being taken off another's. Individuals who consider themselves unattached to any particular practitioner may well still be registered with a family doctor whom they used to consult many years previously. That practitioner will have received an annual capitation fee for the patient whether or not any consultations took place.

Do you need permission to change doctors?

A patient who has recently moved from one area to another, or whose practitioner has moved practice premises, died or retired, can register with another family doctor without any additional formalities, but a patient who has *not* moved home and simply wants to leave one doctor's list and join another's must either obtain written permission from both doctors for the change, or must wait fourteen days after presenting his medical card to the new doctor before the registration will be allowed to go through. Under no circumstances does a patient have to give any reasons for wishing to change doctors.

If patients on the list of a doctor who has retired or died do not notify the Family Practitioner Committee that they wish to join another doctor's list they will automatically be transferred to whichever doctor has taken over the deceased or retired practitioner's responsibilities.

Should a patient decide to leave his doctor's list but then find that it is impossible to find another practitioner prepared to accept him as a patient he can ask the Family Practitioner Committee for help. The FPC will then allocate the patient to a particular doctor in its area and that doctor must provide the patient with care although he may, in due course, ask for the individual to be removed from his list of patients. If that happens the patient must be reallocated.

What happens to your medical records?

Once a patient has changed doctors his medical records must begin the complicated journey from one doctor's filing system to another doctor's filing system. The FPC responsible for the area in which the second doctor practises will write to the FPC for the area in which the first doctor practises and ask for the notes. This FPC will then write to the doctor who has the notes and ask him to return them; when it has the notes the one FPC will send them to the other FPC. The notes will then be sent on to the new doctor. This whole procedure can, and often does, take several months, during which time the patient's new doctor will have to work in ignorance of the patient's past medical history. If, however, the new doctor feels that there is likely to be information of vital importance in those notes he can either contact his own FPC and ask them to expedite the process or contact the patient's first doctor directly for information.

Problems in changing your doctor

In practice there are a number of problems which can make changing doctors difficult.

To begin with there is the undoubted fact that general practitioners are in what might be rather vulgarly called a 'buyer's market' as far as acquiring patients is concerned. The point is that there is a relative shortage of GPs at the moment and a relative glut of patients. Few principals in general practice are actively concerned with increasing the size of their lists since the additional financial rewards for looking after more patients are greatly limited.

In addition it is undoubtedly true that many doctors are suspicious of patients wishing to change doctors while still living in the same area. This suspicion is based on the unjust assumption that if a patient and a doctor have fallen out the falling-out must have been the patient's fault.

It is, I am afraid, up to the patient wishing to make a change to convince the new doctor that the breakdown in the relationship resulted not simply from faults on the patient's part but from a failure on both sides to develop and cement a good relationship. Few doctors would disagree with the suggestion that general practitioners are, by and large, independent, perhaps even slightly eccentric on occasions, and that therefore a breakdown in a relationship may well have been caused by faults on both sides.

Some patients feel that before joining a new doctor's list they are entitled to 'try him out' and to make a preliminary visit to assess his capabilities both as a doctor and as a human being. This is entirely reasonable and if a patient is moving into a new area there need be no problems since the doctor can see the patient as a temporary resident and neither patient nor doctor need be embarrassed by any failure to consummate the encounter. If a patient who has not moved into a new area wishes to change doctors the problem is slightly trickier since the rules of the NHS preclude a GP from giving advice or information to another doctor's patient except where, in an emergency, the patient's own doctor has not been available.

Under these circumstances there are two possibilities. Either the patient can leave his own doctor and then visit the new doctor and explain that he wishes to have a trial consultation, or he can remain on his own doctor's list and visit the new doctor purely to study the facilities and examine the doctor as a suitable candidate. I'm afraid that neither venture is likely to prove popular and the GP honoured by the examination is unlikely to accept the would-be patient. The most dignified way to make the change must surely be to decide in advance on a doctor likely to prove suitable, to visit him and ask to be accepted on his list. If the doctor says no for any reason, the patient still has a doctor. If the doctor says yes, the change can go through with or without the patient's previous doctor being consulted.

When a doctor decides to remove a patient from his list

So far I have dealt exclusively with what happens when a patient wants to change doctors. There are of course also occasions when a doctor decides that he no longer wishes to provide a particular patient with medical care. This freedom is sometimes opposed by militant patient organizations, by politicians who really ought to know better, and by social workers and journalists who have little conception of what the responsibility of a doctor-patient relationship involves for the practitioner concerned.

Very few doctors take advantage of this freedom more than once or twice a year and only then when they find themselves unable to offer unemotional, honest medical care any longer.

There are a number of reasons why a doctor may feel that he can no longer accept an individual as a patient or accept full responsibility for that patient's well-being. If, for example, a patient has been particularly rude or aggressive the doctor may feel that the relationship has broken down and is beyond repair. If the patient has made demands upon the doctor's time which have seemed unreasonable (and which may, for example, have included out-of-hours calls for routine problems) the doctor may feel that looking after this one patient makes life so unpleasant as to threaten not only the doctor's own health but also that of the other patients for whom he is responsible.

When a doctor decides to remove a patient from his list he simply has to inform the Family Practitioner Committee. He does not have to give any reason for the removal. The FPC will then write to the patient concerned inviting him to register with another local doctor. If the patient cannot find another doctor able or willing to accept him as a patient then the FPC will allocate him to a particular practice which must, temporarily at least, provide medical cover. Particularly troublesome patients are sometimes passed around from doctor to doctor with each local practitioner serving a three-month sentence.

Incidentally, just as some patients now insist on vetting doctors so some doctors insist on vetting would-be patients. This is done in an attempt to avoid getting into the sort of situation I have described above.

Choosing or changing your doctor: points to remember

We have seen that choosing or changing your doctor may be simple enough in theory but that in practice it can be difficult. There are, however, several fairly obvious ways to avoid trouble.

1 When moving into a new area, by all means take your time choosing a new doctor, but do make arrangements as soon as possible after your move. Do not wait until you are ill.

2 When you have selected a likely doctor ask to see him as a temporary resident. This can be done by simply turning up if the surgeries are open or by telephoning to make an appointment. Even if you do not need any regular supplies of pills (such as the contraceptive pill) it should not be too difficult to find some member of the family with a realistic symptom.

3 Once you register with a doctor, treat him with the same respect that you expect from him. He has a duty to treat you with courtesy and care and you have the same duty to him. Try to begin a new relationship with a doctor in an optimistic mood. If you expect him to be awful, he probably will be.

4 If you find a practitioner in a group practice difficult to get on with there is not usually any difficulty in seeing another practitioner in the same practice. You do not necessarily have to change from one doctor's list to another. Whenever possible, however, you should try to see the same doctor in order to build up a relationship. Remember that it will not always be possible to see your own doctor if you request an urgent appointment.

Patient participation

Eight years ago the first patient participation group was started. Today there are thirty-two such groups in Britain – most of them started not by patients but by doctors.

The aim is for a committee of patients to help run the practice, to advise on ways to improve the service available and to provide the doctor with a supply of information from his patients. It is, after all, a fact of life that most patients are reluctant to offer their doctor direct criticism although they may be ready to make adverse comments at a safe distance. The patient participation group can provide individuals with a certain amount of anonymity.

It is too early to say whether or not these groups have a useful future. At the moment it seems likely that the only doctors who are prepared to listen to patients' representatives are the ones who least need advice.

Ethical dilemmas

The ethical, legal, moral, contractual and social responsibilities, duties and commitments of general practitioners are too many to number here, let alone discuss in detail. And to complicate matters further there are disputes, controversies and dilemmas associated with just about every single responsibility, duty and commitment.

Since Hammurabi first wrote his Code and Hippocrates compiled his Oath, doctors, philosophers and lawyers have struggled with the many ethical dilemmas associated with medical practice. Today the advances made by scientists and technologists have made the ethical dilemmas even more complicated, and have added to the number of problems by creating new possibilities and new concepts. The increasing importance of the bureaucracy within medicine, the rising importance of the state and the revolution against doctor control and patient dependence have all led to changes in the expectations of both patients and doctors, and to the development of a whole range of new political, social and economic mechanisms designed to weaken the importance of the doctor-patient relationship and the value of mutual trust. Organizations representing doctors and associations representing patients have struggled to prepare comprehensive accounts of the dilemmas that there are and to provide puzzled practitioners with advice, support and direction. So far all such attempts have failed and the many questions that have to be faced remain unanswered.

Not even the basic rights of patients and doctors have been properly evaluated and there is as yet no agreement as to the rights of patients to have good health, to obtain treatment, to be told the truth, to be allowed to die or to be kept alive. Nor is there any agreement on whether doctors should provide patients with what they need or with what they want, or on the responsibilities of patients to care for their own bodies or to listen to the advice offered by their physicians.

Indeed, from the evidence available it seems unlikely that it will ever be possible to draw up strict rules and regulations governing all eventualities and capable of ensuring that all health care professionals will follow strictly defined obligations on all occasions.

A better alternative is surely for doctors to understand and accept their obligations to patients and to agree to behave purely and simply in the interest of their patients. It is, after all, the role of the general practitioner to guide his patients through the maze of health care bureaucracy and to protect them from the technological excesses of specialists, who may be so involved in the diagnosis and treatment of particular disease processes that they fail to see the patient as an individual human being, entitled to be treated with respect and consideration.

For general practitioners to be able to act in this way it is vital for patients to be prepared to trust them. Such cooperation must inevitably lead to a reduction in the emphasis on patients' and doctors' rights.

Plato argued that physicians should take patients and their families into their confidence, that they should discuss things in a scientific way, that they should learn from their patients and only provide treatment after winning their patients' support and persuading them to comply with their recommendations.

Plato's ideas on this subject are still of value and it seems to me that the very many ethical dilemmas that exist today (a few of which are discussed on the following pages) will only be solved when confidence and trust are restored to the doctor-patient relationship. Neither can be obtained as a right by either side in the partnership, but both can and should be earned.

Abortion

The law in Britain allows doctors to terminate pregnancies as long as certain conditions are met. Two doctors must see the patient and they must agree that the conditions laid down in the 1967 Abortion Act have been satisfied. Since the conditions allow doctors to recommend terminations where they feel that continuing with the pregnancy would be a hazard to either the mental or the physical welfare of the patient this means that in practice abortion is available on demand in certain areas of the country. The most relevant phrase on the green form – Certificate A/Form HSA1 – which doctors must sign before an abortion can be performed is: 'The continuation of the pregnancy would involve risk to the life of the pregnant woman, or of injury to the physical or mental health of the pregnant woman or any existing children of her family greater than if the pregnancy were terminated.'

The availability of abortion under the National Health Service varies from area to area. In some parts of Britain NHS abortions are almost impossible to obtain. In other parts of Britain there are very few problems for women seeking free abortions.

The comparative ease with which abortions can be obtained in Britain is opposed by certain religious groups who argue that the unborn foetus has a right to life. A relatively small but vociferous group of doctors are members of these groups and for their own personal reasons will refuse to provide patients with advice or information about abortions. It is therefore important that any woman preparing to discuss abortion with her own GP should be aware of his or her opinions. A brief telephone conversation with the receptionist may elicit the required information.

Whether or not doctors have a personal right to refuse to co-operate with women seeking abortions is as contentious an issue as whether or not abortion is ever justified.

As a practical point I would like to suggest that all doctors who disapprove of abortion for their own personal reasons should be prepared to make their feelings known to their own patients (perhaps by a small notice in the waiting room). This would enable patients seeking abortions to avoid embarrassing themselves or their doctors by making requests which offend. Similarly a public statement detailing a doctor's attitudes towards contraception might ease another potential source of friction.

Where a patient's general practitioner is unwilling to provide advice, the local branch of the British Pregnancy Advisory Service (see p. 176 or local telephone directory) should be able to help.

In recent years the problem of abortion has become even more complicated with the introduction of amniocentesis (see p. 186) and foetal sex-testing kits. It is now known that women have obtained abortions because the sex of their unborn babies was not acceptable. The social and economic consequences of this trend are far-reaching and will undoubtedly tax the minds of all who are interested in the subject.

Advertising

Traditionally there are strict rules in Britain which forbid doctors from advertising. These rules, given teeth by the General Medical Council, make it an offence for a doctor to have a name plate that is too large, a telephone directory entry that is too comprehensive or a passion for personal publicity which can be shown to have any effect on the number of patients seeking his help.

In recent years the rules have been relaxed and today it is considered reasonable for a practitioner to allow himself to be named on television, radio or in newspapers or magazines as long as there is no question that he is trying to attract patients to himself. The General Medical Council points out that it is an offence if a doctor sanctions any publication which draws attention to his own special skills.

Incidentally, in America, as a result of an order from the Federal Trade Commission, the American Medical Association has now dropped its long-standing ban on doctors' advertising.

Artificial insemination

The legal and ethical problems associated with artificial insemination seem endless. The precise nature of the problem involved varies according to the source of the sperm used and the place where fertilization occurs.

It is up to lawyers rather than doctors to decide whether or not a marriage has been consummated, whether the resulting infant is legitimate, what rights the biological father has and what rights the woman's husband has if the sperm has come from a donor. The preservation of human sperm in sperm banks, the use of celebrity sperm, the developments in the field of test-tube babies and the questions of whether or not artificial insemination constitutes legal adultery are other problems which must worry the lawyers.

Doctors, on the other hand, have the responsibility of ensuring that, where a donor's sperm is used, there is no history of genetic or infectious disease, and that all parties involved are physically and mentally capable of coping with the inevitable stresses.

Confidentiality

The problem of confidentiality is perhaps the most important single ethical dilemma involving general practitioners today. It is, after all, completely reasonable for patients to expect that the intimate details they reveal in the doctor's surgery will remain intimate. Patients who do not have faith that their secrets will be kept will be unlikely to trust doctors with secrets any more, and without access to intimate details and secrets doctors would be incapable of making diagnoses.

When doctors simply talked to their patients and scribbled a few semi-legible notes down on bits of card the problem of confidentiality was relatively simple. The major threat was posed by judges and lawyers who have always opposed the right of doctors to maintain patient confidentiality but who, as far as I know, have never actually had the courage to insist on doctors' giving away information that they did not want to give away. (The law in Britain states quite clearly that if ordered to do so by a court of law a doctor must divulge confidential information but in practice I do not know of any case where a doctor has been forced to give away information that he felt he ought to keep secret.)

Today there are three far more practical threats to the principle of confidentiality: the increase in the number of paramedical workers and administrative aides involved in the health care business; changes in the way that medical information is now stored; and the increasing number of organizations (both private and public) which claim access to medical records.

In the days when the GP made his own notes and wrote his own letters, and the number of people involved in health care was relatively small, there were, of course, few problems about information leaking out. Even when doctors began employing receptionists and secretaries the risks were acceptably slight. Today, however, the doctor and his immediate, personal staff make up only a small part of the army of people concerned with the provision of medical care. In addition to nurses, chiropodists, physiotherapists, health visitors and opticians (all of whom are bound by ethical codes to maintain secrecy) there are now endless numbers of social workers and health service administrators who are not bound by any effective code of practice. Some of these workers have specifically declared their disapproval of the principle of patient confidentiality, and have announced that they would be prepared to divulge confidential information to lawyers, school teachers, policemen and others who have no direct interest in the physical or mental welfare of the individual concerned and who may, indeed, be directly concerned with doing that individual harm.

The problem of the way in which medical information is stored has, of course, been made considerably more serious by the fact that an increasing number of medical authorities are using computer storage systems for medical information. As has been shown many times, computers may not be capable of exhibiting original wisdom or stupidity, but they can magnify human wisdom and human stupidity. In addition, as many industrial companies have discovered to their cost and embarrassment, computers are relatively easy to burgle. Even sophisticated computer equipment, intended to protect highly valuable information, has been badly stung by schoolboy enthusiasts with guile, patience and basic training.

The advocates of computer storage systems argue that the information can be protected by preparing rules about who can and who cannot have access to the computer tapes but none of the protective devices so far developed has proved foolproof and no system of voluntary control can possibly exclude those who are determined to obtain secret information.

In Britain, where doctors have for some time been conscious that computer records could be too easily used by the state, the Medical Research Council has made detailed recommendations designed to guide those planning to make use of computerized medical records. One of the most important recommendations of the Medical Research Council is that only a physician should have the responsibility to decide the extent to which computer records should be made available. Unfortunately there is, I fear, too much evidence to suggest that not all physicians are always motivated to act entirely in the interests of individual patients. There is certainly no evidence to suggest that physicians involved in pure research work or employed as administrators would be at all reluctant to make information available to organizations and departments concerned more with public welfare than with private rights.

The question of which organizations should be entitled to obtain access to medical records has become more and more difficult to answer in recent years as an increasing number of people have recognized the value of medical information. For example, many industrial and commercial concerns regularly and routinely extract confidential information from sick notes originally intended to be used for national insurance purposes only. It is common for personnel officers employed by large companies to demand and expect to be given private information about employees. Many lawyers preparing cases for the civil courts expect to be provided with information and the police often demand confidential information as if it were a right.

In addition, there are the insurance companies that write to general practitioners and ask for information about patients' past medical histories. It is true that patients will usually have signed release forms giving their doctors permission to release the information but few patients realize the extent of the information required and there is no guarantee that once an insurance company has obtained information it will not make that information available to other companies through computer records or printed reports. Since the information requested by insurance companies may include information that has not been divulged to the patient the risks associated with the sale of information in this way may be considerable.

In practice general practitioners deal with the problem of confidentiality in many different ways. Some are careful not to divulge confidential information to anyone and will refuse to accept fees from insurance companies requesting information even when those companies have obtained written permission from patients, arguing that only rarely has the patient been aware that he is being asked to give permission for such information to be divulged and that even then he may have no idea of what sort of information is likely to be made available or the use that may be made of it.

Some doctors, on the other hand, are fairly free with information and are happy to make confidential notes available without any restrictions. Some general practitioners, when asked for information from government departments are swayed by the argument that the Secretary of State owns all NHS medical records and that the practitioner is therefore not entitled to restrict the availability of the information on these records. In fact I rather suspect that although the medical record cards belong to the Secretary of State the ink and writing upon them do in fact belong to the doctor or doctors responsible for actually making the notes.

Consent

Patients are often invited to give written consent before allowing doctors to perform tests or operative precedures. It is important that any patient preparing to sign such a consent form should take time to read carefully what rights he is signing away. Before operative procedures, for example, patients are frequently expected to give surgeons permission to carry out any procedures found necessary. This may sound frightening but the reasons for the blanket consent is simple: if the surgeon finds something that needs dealing with while the patient is under the anaesthetic he cannot proceed unless he has written consent. To do otherwise would be to risk a charge of assault. So, for example, a surgeon performing an operation on a woman with a breast lump may ask for permission to perform radical surgery should the lump prove to be malignant. The alternative is to perform an investigation, wake the patient, obtain permission and then proceed with the necessary surgery at a later date.

Many doctors recognize that obtaining genuine, realistic consent from patients is not as easy as it sounds. For one thing patients are usually frightened before any operative procedure and rarely in a position to judge whether or not a particular test should or should not be done. In addition there are extra pressures which may arise as a result of a patient's concept of what is expected of him. For example, a potential kidney donor, bone marrow donor or blood donor may feel that to refuse permission for an operation that they do not need but which may prove beneficial to some other individual might be considered churlish.

There are occasions, of course, when a patient's consent cannot be obtained. For example Jehovah's Witnesses sometimes refuse to give permission for their children to receive necessary blood transfusions on religious grounds, taking advantage of the fact that no doctor is entitled to carry out any procedure on a child under the age of 16 without the parents' consent (see also Contraception). Official policy, however, is that in an emergency medical practitioners are entitled to perform necessary procedures even where parents have deliberately witheld permission.

Finally, there are those mentally ill patients who are not capable of giving permission for treatment to be instigated. Where doctors believe that patients are likely to be a genuine danger to themselves or to others they may invoke the 1959 Mental Health Act and arrange for patients to be admitted to hospital (see p. 148).

Contraception

The provision of contraception is in itself a controversial subject since there are many who feel that all artificial forms of contraception should be opposed on religious grounds. Because of personal beliefs there are some doctors in general practice who refuse to offer contraceptive advice to any of their patients. In theory these doctors should always recommend alternative practitioners since there is no real justification for a doctor to allow his own religious beliefs to affect his patients in this way, but, unfortunately, there are a number of practitioners who not only refuse to provide contraceptive advice but also refuse to countenance it. Occasionally these practitioners may impose specific moral judgments but be prepared to refer married women, or women over a certain age, to other doctors.

Where this problem does exist there are usually other practitioners willing and able to offer advice. There may, for example, be another member of the practice with more liberal ideas or there may be a local family planning clinic. Where neither of these sources is available a patient is entitled to visit any practitioner working within the National Health Service or in private practice and to ask for help and advice. Should the patient's own doctor object to any action that is taken the patient may well be wise to consider changing to a more amenable practice.

The most controversial aspect of contraception has in recent years concerned the provision of contraceptive advice to girls under the age of sixteen. A number of parents and practitioners have joined together to form active pressure groups designed to oppose the provision of any sort of contraceptive advice to girls under the age of sixteen but in particular to oppose the provision of advice to girls whose parents do not approve or whose permission has not been obtained.

The argument sometimes put forward by those who oppose the provision of contraception to the under-sixteens is that no girl can legally have intercourse under that age and enabling her to do so without risk is in some way aiding or abetting her partner to commit an offence. In addition it is argued that girls under the age of sixteen are unlikely to be able to remember to take contraceptive pills, that making the pill available encourages promiscuity and that making the pill available without the parents having given consent is in some way detracting from the rights of the parents. One doctor who opposes the provision of contraception to girls under sixteen has reportedly argued that there is no such thing as confidentiality between a child and a doctor but that a confidential relationship relating to the child can only exist between the doctor and the parents.

The Department of Health and Social Security has issued a memorandum offering guidance to practitioners in which it is suggested that doctors should always try and persuade children to involve their parents or guardians but it is admitted that under some circumstances parental involvement cannot be obtained and that, when that is the case, to refuse to offer contraceptive advice would not be in the child's interest.

Those who continue to provide contraceptive advice to the under-sixteens argue that there is no physical reason for not doing so, that the current law simply reflects social convention and that, since girls under sixteen are old enough to get pregnant without their parents, they should surely be entitled to obtain contraceptive advice on their own. It has been argued that, if girls go to a family doctor for contraception and do not want their parents to know, there has been a breakdown in communication between parents and child. It is said that it is because they recognize the existence of a communication failure (which is in itself a reflection on their status as parents) that parents object so vehemently.

On purely ethical grounds it is difficult to understand why a fifteen-and-a-half year old girl is less entitled to have a confidential relationship with a medical practitioner than a sixteen year-old girl.

Girls under sixteen who have difficulty in obtaining advice from a family doctor may seek help from a family planning clinic or Brook clinic. In addition it should be pointed out that there are practitioners who are prepared to prescribe the contraceptive pill to under-age girls for therapeutic reasons (it is sometimes used to control painful or irregular periods) while appreciating that the pill is in fact being used for another purpose as well.

Delegation

It is a doctor's responsibility to ensure that any individual who is allowed to attend to patients on his behalf or with his permission is qualified to do so. This means that before allowing a district nurse or practice nurse to carry out any procedure the doctor must be satisfied that the nurse is capable of carrying it out. It also means that the physician is responsible for ensuring that any deputizing service he employs or any locum he hires is competent.

A patient who believes that anyone operating on behalf of his practitioner is not competent should make this clear to the doctor concerned.

Strictly speaking, GPs are not allowed to refer patients to individuals who are not officially recognized as members of a supplementary medical profession. In practice, however, many GPs are willing to cooperate unofficially with specific named individuals working outside the official profession or the confines of the health service. An open unaddressed 'referral' letter is sometimes a suitable way of satisfying medical etiquette without failing the patient.

Dishonesty

Doctors who are found guilty of any form of dishonesty are likely to find themselves before the General Medical Council. Under certain circumstances doctors can be charged with fraud if they provide patients whom they have not seen with sick notes.

It is this combination of facts which make many family doctors wary of handing out sick notes as freely as patients might sometimes like.

Euthanasia

The whole question of suicide, euthanasia and mercy killings has been a subject for much public discussion in recent years. The wider availability of complex life-support machinery means that today doctors can, in theory at least, keep people alive long after they would have died if certain basic functions had not been taken over artificially. The availability of antibiotics means that many elderly people who might have died peacefully of pneumonia can be kept alive, whether they want to live or not. And the progress in surgery means that many congenitally deformed babies, who might otherwise have died, can be kept alive even though they will never be capable of living an independent life.

Some doctors argue that it is a medical duty always to strive to keep patients alive for as long as possible – whatever the consequences and whatever the physical or mental state of the patient may be. Others claim that it is a doctor's duty to resist the temptation to strive 'officiously' to keep patients alive when they no longer have any opportunity to live a life which could be described as meaningful. And there is a small but vociferous group who argue that under some circumstances a doctor is right to take life and to make death as painless as possible. The ethical and philosophical arguments are often coloured and confused by the accompanying social and economic problems.

Although it is difficult to generalize I believe that most doctors in practice in Britain try to steer a course between extremes. The majority of practitioners believe that it is always right to deal with a patient's pain, even when the nature and quantity of pain-killing drugs required may endanger life or hasten death. It is also widely believed that patients have a right to die in peace and with dignity, and for this reason there are GPs who try to keep the terminally ill at home for as long as possible. It is common for practitioners to absolve themselves of direct responsibility for the early demise of a patient by handing over responsibility to God. So, for example, a doctor looking after a dying ninety-year-old who has a painful terminal illness complicated by a chest infection may not insist that antibiotics be given by injection when the patient fails to swallow oral medication. And, similarly, a doctor may not insist that a newly born baby with a serious congenital defect be fed artificially if the baby is failing to feed naturally.

These are difficult questions to which there are no final answers. Most good doctors ask themselves one simple question before making such decisions: 'What would I like done if I were the patient or if the patient were a close relative of mine?'

Experimentation

Human experimentation may be divided into three categories. First, there are the procedures which doctors try out on themselves. Second, there are the experiments performed on healthy volunteers (students, drug company employees and prisoners) where there is no expectation that the volunteer will benefit directly from the experiment. And, finally, there are the experiments carried out on patients which involve the use of some diagnostic or therapeutic procedure that may or may not prove to be of value. It is this third category of experiments which concerns the general practitioner's patients most clearly.

The first point to be made about this type of experimentation is that it is sometimes extremely difficult to decide where normal procedures end and experiments begin. Every patient is different, and there are variations in the ways in which all patients respond to procedures and treatments. In a sense, therefore, whenever a doctor writes a prescription he is beginning a new experiment.

On a number of specific occasions, however, it is clear from the outset that the treatment is experimental – for example, when a new drug is being tested on a limited number of patients before being made available to all doctors and all patients. This is happening more and more frequently today, since a growing number of drug company advisers are becoming aware that tests conducted by hospital doctors on hospital patients under hospital conditions are of limited significance if the drugs involved are eventually going to be given by GPs to patients in the community.

Unfortunately, although it is true that a number of GPs are well able to conduct simple drug trials successfully, it is also a fact that some GPs are today conducting drug trials without a true understanding of the associated hazards. It is not unknown for drug companies to offer GPs money or equipment to take part in drug-testing programmes, and I am not convinced that under those circumstances the patients are always provided with the appropriate degree of extra medical care.

It is usual for practitioners contemplating trials of this kind to inform their patients that a new product is being tested and to ask if they are willing to take part in the tests. Any patient who is not willing should say so straight away.

Personally, I do not believe that any patient should be asked to take part in a trial until a reasonable attempt has been made to control that patient's symptoms with all other available and fully tested products. Then the patient should be warned that unusual side effects may occur and that any abnormal reaction should be reported immediately to the doctor conducting the trial. The doctor should be willing to give the patient his own home telephone number if a trial is being conducted since the practitioner's own partners or deputizing service may not be aware of the trial's purpose or any associated hazards. The patient should be checked at least once a week in the surgery.

Incidentally, any patient who is given a full supply of a drug without an accompanying prescription may be taking part in a trial of a new product and should check before accepting the supply of drugs.

Patients' rights

Although the law defines the responsibilities of doctors quite strictly it does not define the rights of patients with anything like as much precision. As doctor-patient relationships have soured, and as patients have become better educated, more interested and better able to judge for themselves the advantages and disadvantages associated with certain diagnostic procedures and forms of treatment, the number of patients demanding certain specific rights and refusing to allow doctors to dictate to them has increased. There are a number of areas which seem particularly to attract attention and cause concern. I will deal with three of them here.

First, there is the question of whether or not patients should have access to their own medical records. Those who support this argument claim that it is a patient's basic right to have access to anything written about himself and that the law which forbids a patient the right to study his own notes is unjust. It is claimed that doctors frequently label patients, and that the labels they use (hypochondriac, neurotic, and so on) may prejudice a patient's future medical advisers. It is also argued that some doctors write derogatory notes in medical records ('a bloody nuisance', 'always moaning' and so on) and that these notes may also prejudice future medical treatment.

On the other hand, those who oppose the right of patients to see their own notes argue that if patients had access to notes then doctors would be unwilling to record information that seemed subjective but might be of value. Also, they say, notes about social circumstances and about relatives are likely to be omitted.

More important, perhaps, is the argument that if patients are to have access to their own notes doctors will be unwilling to record differential diagnoses. For example, a patient with a particular set of symptoms may have any one of a number of disorders. In his preliminary notes the doctor may record suggestions such as 'cancer' or 'leukaemia' simply because these are diseases which must be excluded. Seeing these diseases recorded in his notes may cause a patient to panic.

Indeed, the whole question of whether or not patients should always be told the diagnosis even when the diagnosis is beyond doubt is another subject of concern. Some patients insist that they do want to be told, others insist that they do not want to be told. Some need to know the truth; some need to be supported with lies. Deciding who to tell and who not to tell is a problem that doctors face regularly. The argument about whether or not they should take that decision themselves is one which will go on for some time.

Another important area of patients' rights is pregnancy and childbirth. Some doctors today are unwilling to allow their patients to have babies at home. They claim that the facilities in hospitals are better, the dangers at home are much greater if anything goes wrong and that their own training and practical experience are not good enough to enable them to take the responsibility for home deliveries. Patients, on the other hand, argue that statistics show home childbirth to be safe, that giving birth is a natural event and not the culmination of an illness, that hospital practitioners are more likely to induce a birth, and that they are prepared to accept any risks which may exist.

This, too, is a subject of concern which will continue to be debated for some years, but meanwhile any woman whose own doctor is not prepared to allow her to have a home confinement is entitled to ask another practitioner to look after her. She need not necessarily change doctors to do this. In most areas there is still usually one practitioner with an interest in home confinement who has the necessary skills and experience to cope with most of the problems that can arise.

A third major problem area involves the provision of contraceptive advice to women over the age of thirty-five. There have in recent years been many studies of the risks associated with taking the contraceptive pill, and most of these have shown that the danger of circulatory troubles increases considerably with the age of the woman concerned. In view of this fact many doctors now routinely ask patients in their mid-thirties to consider alternative forms of contraception. The woman of thirty-five, they claim, may well remain fertile for another fifteen years and providing her with the contraceptive pill for the whole of that period must pose a genuine health risk.

The patients concerned will, however, sometimes argue that if they are willing to take the risk they should be allowed to do so. It is the doctor's duty, they claim, to offer advice and information and then to respect the patient's wishes. Unfortunately, the legal responsibilities of practitioners are not so clear cut and many doctors fear that they could face heavy legal damages if a patient died or was incapacitated as a result of her taking the pill at a time when statistics show that the risks are appreciably increased.

All these problems and many others will undoubtedly continue to cause controversy and excite discussion for years to come. There is little doubt that many patients view medical professionals as members of a 'service' profession and themselves as consumers. The problem is that although they want consumer rights patients are not always prepared to take on any of the physician's ethical or legal responsibilities.

Sexual offences

Doctors, like all members of the community, can be charged with indecent exposure or rape if the appropriate charges are made and the suitable evidence is provided. If a charge of either kind is found proven in a court of law then the practitioner will almost certainly find himself before the General Medical Council, whether or not the victim was a patient.

Practitioners are always expected to behave with propriety when dealing with patients and practitioners suspected of using their professional position to further a relationship of any kind with a patient would have to defend themselves before the General Medical Council. However, if a patient has been a willing partner in a relationship the General Medical Council is less likely to be interested in any subsequent complaint.

Sterilization

Sterilization is a form of permanent contraception favoured by many couples. Either the male or the female may be sterilized and most British surgeons will usually insist that the partner gives permission together with the prospective patient, although in law each partner is entitled to be sterilized without the other's consent. In addition, surgeons will usually want both partners to appreciate that although sterilization operations can occasionally be successfully reversed it is wiser to consider a sterilization operation as permanent. Some surgeons ask patients to consider whether or not they would want more children if, for example, their children died or they remarried. Many patients then reasonably point out that children cannot be replaced. Occasionally surgeons will perform sterilization operations on unmarried individuals or on one member of a childless married couple when it is clear that the individual or couple concerned do not want to have children at all.

Sterilization of any individual without his or her consent is usually considered to be a violation of civil rights and a breach of the law.

Violence

Practitioners found guilty of assault in a court of law are likely to find themselves explaining their behaviour to the General

Medical Council. The members of the appropriate committee may be particularly disapproving if the victim of the assault is a patient or another practitioner, although practitioners are allowed to defend themselves against attacks by disturbed or violent patients.

Making a complaint about a GP

In the course of a single year general practitioners meet patients about 250 million times. On each one of these occasions there is a good chance that the patient will feel emotionally taut, vulnerable, dependent, frightened and suspicious. There is also a good chance that the doctor he meets will feel bored, tired and depressed by the pressure of work and the extent of his responsibility.

Add to these facts the undeniable truths that GPs have a considerable amount of power (literally the power of life and death in some circumstances), that there is very often no chance at all for the patient to maintain any active choice over the type of treatment he is offered, that there is an inbuilt imbalance between the professional and the consumer because of the professional's technical knowledge and the consumer's ignorance, and that much medical work and many medical decisions have to be made very quickly without time for discussion or reflection, and it is hardly surprising that on occasion patients feel the need to grumble or complain about their doctors. Indeed, given all these circumstances it is perhaps surprising that GPs remain as popular as they do and that the number of active complaints made is as small as it is.

On many occasions the patient is probably content to grumble, appreciating that the doctor's apparent boorishness is a human failing rather than a professional one and that there is little point in making a serious complaint. (The complaint would, in any case, be dismissed since there is no machinery through which a patient may make a complaint about a doctor's manners. But then there is no machinery for a doctor to complain about a rude patient.)

The top ten grumbles about GPs

1 The doctor is rude or bad mannered

2 The doctor's receptionist is rude or bad mannered

3 A home visit was either refused or there was an unreasonable delay

4 Inadequate treatment or examination was provided

5 The appointments system does not work satisfactorily

6 The doctor failed to make an appropriate referral to a specialist or to other health service facilities

7 It is impossible to contact the doctor by telephone

8 The doctor failed to provide a needed medical certificate

9 The doctor's deputizing service for emergency calls is not satisfactory

10 The doctor does not provide an appointment system

Because only complaints about a doctor failing to observe his Terms of Service merit investigation by an FPC the top two grumbles do not qualify for the official complaints procedure. The same is true of grumbles 5, 7, 9 and 10 unless the difficulty grumbled about actually constitutes a breach of the practitioner's Terms of Service.

When the problem is more important, however, and a complaint is seriously considered it is vital to know exactly how complaints can be filed. In the section which follows I have described the three main ways in which individuals may make formal complaints about family doctors: through the Family Practitioner Committee, the law courts, and the General Medical Council.

It is perhaps worthwhile pointing out that the British Medical Association is a doctors' union which, among other things, exists to further the economic interests of the medical profession. It does not represent all members of the medical profession and there is no point at all in making a complaint about a practitioner to any of its officers or committees.

The Health Services Commissioner (see p. 120) is not usually concerned with complaints made about general practitioners.

Making a complaint to the FPC

A complaint about a GP may be made to the local Family Practitioner Committee by a patient, a patient's relative, someone representing the patient, someone authorized by the patient, someone acting on behalf of a deceased patient, by officials of the health service or by the Secretary of State. However, if a complaint is made more than 8 weeks after the incident that is the subject of the complaint either the GP concerned or the Secretary of State must give permission for the complaint to be heard.

When to complain to the FPC

When making a complaint to a Family Practitioner Committee it is important to realize that the Committee is only interested in allegations which involve a suggested breach of the practitioner's Terms of Service – in other words his contract with the Secretary of State. The FPC will have nothing to do with a complaint that a doctor has made a clinical error or has not made the right diagnosis.

It is also important to remember that doctors in general practice are only expected to maintain standards which ordinary, reasonable GPs could be expected to maintain. In other words, the FPC will not support a complaint that a general practitioner did not do a test for Von Tootree's disease if there has only been one case of Von Tootree's disease in Northern Europe in the last twenty-five years. In practice, there are frequent disagreements about what an ordinary, competent GP might or might not be expected to do. In general those doctors who work for the DHSS and who never see patients tend to expect more than those doctors who have active experience of the day-to-day pressures in general practice.

The procedure

Once a complaint has been made it will be passed to the Administrator of the local FPC. He may feel that the complaint is a fairly trivial one and that it may be possible to clear up the problem by talking to both patient and doctor. If, however, the complaint is more serious or if the patient is not willing to consider an informal approach to the problem, then a formal report will be submitted to the lay chairman of the Medical Services Committee. This is a subcommittee of the FPC and includes doctors and lay members.

The chairman will then have the duty to decide whether or not there are true grounds for complaint. If he feels that the complaint is not covered by the GP's Terms of Service he will order that the complaint be dismissed. The person who has made the complaint does, however, have the right to appeal to the Secretary of State if this happens.

Otherwise, the next step is for the complaint to be heard in private by the whole of the Medical Services Committee. A considerable amount of time may elapse between the making of a complaint and its being heard by the committee and it is not unknown for this time to be as much as two years. In practice the delay usually causes more heartache to the practitioner than to the complainant.

101

The Medical Services Committee has no power to insist that witnesses appear and does not allow either the doctor or the patient to hire professional advocates. Friends may accompany the complainant and the defendant and may speak on their behalf.

When it has heard evidence from both sides the Committee may either dismiss the complaint or uphold it. If the case is dismissed the complainant may appeal. If the complaint is upheld the committee may decide that no action is needed, that the doctor must be warned, that a sum of money should be witheld from his next NHS cheque or, in exceptional circumstances, that his name should be removed from the list of approved health service GPs. Whatever the committee decides is appropriate, the papers dealing with the hearing will be sent to the DHSS and studied by civil servants for final approval. If a complaint is upheld a doctor may appeal against any sentence which may be passed.

The local FPC address can be obtained by looking in the local telephone directory or by studying your medical card FP4.

Complaints about dentists, opticians and pharmacists

Family Practitioner Committees are also responsible for the services provided by dentists, opticians and pharmacists. Complaints about services provided by professionals in these groups should be made directly to the Administrator of the local FPC who will, if necessary, pass the complaint on to the chairman of the appropriate subcommittee. (There are three subcommittees working alongside the Medical Services Committee.)

In addition, complaints about the activities of dentists, opticians and pharmacists can be submitted to the General Dental Council, the General Optical Council and the Pharmaceutical Society of Great Britain. (The addresses appear on pp. 168, 169 and 170 respectively.)

For the sake of completeness I should perhaps add that complaints about nurses should be submitted to the General Nursing Council (see p. 168).

The five most important grounds for making a complaint about a GP to the Family Practitioner Committee

1 You feel that your doctor has not provided you with necessary treatment. For example, you may have been refused an appointment when you felt that your condition was urgent. The relevant clause in the GP's contract reads: 'A practitioner is required to render to his patients all proper and necessary treatment.'

2 You believe that your GP should have referred you to a hospital specialist. The relevant clause reads: 'If the condition of the patient is such as to require treatment which is not within the scope of the practitioner's obligations under these terms of service but such treatment is, to the knowledge of the practitioner, available as part of the hospital and specialist services, the practitioner shall inform the patient of the fact and . . . take all necessary steps to enable him to receive such treatment.'

3 You think that your doctor should have visited you at home. The relevant clause is: 'A practitioner is required to visit and treat a patient whose condition so requires at any place where under the terms of his application for the inclusion in the medical list . . . he is under an obligation to visit such a patient.'

4 Your doctor has charged you for a certificate which you think you should not have been charged for. The relevant clause is: 'A practitioner is required to issue to his patients or their personal representatives free of charge the certificates prescribed in Schedule 5 to these regulations.' (This includes national insurance sick notes but not sick notes required by employers.)

5 You think your doctor's surgery or waiting room is unsuitable. The relevant clause is: 'A practitioner is required to provide proper and sufficient surgery and waiting room accommodation for his patients.'

Making a complaint about a private GP

There is no point in making a complaint to a Family Practitioner Committee about the activities of a medical practitioner in private practice. Complaints may, however, still be made through the law courts or to the General Medical Council.

Legal action: when to sue

The traditional way for a patient to make a complaint felt or to obtain redress is for him to sue. To do this successfully a patient must prove that his doctor has failed to exercise reasonable skill and care and that he (the patient) has suffered measurable damage as a result. Medical practitioners will only be found guilty of negligence when it can be shown that they have fallen short of the standards expected of reasonably skilful medical professionals.

In practice, for a case of negligence to succeed, it must be shown that a doctor does not possess the skills he might be expected to possess, or that he did not act with sufficient care when applying his skills, or that he did not act on the basis of honest faith and use good judgment.

It is not negligent to make the wrong diagnosis if everything possible has been done, but it is negligent to make the wrong diagnosis as a result of inadequate care. The doctor who removes a patient's leg without ensuring that he is amputating the correct leg will undoubtedly be found guilty of negligence, as will the doctor who fails to check that a patient can safely take a drug known to be responsible for allergy reactions in some patients. It is negligent to leave instruments inside a patient or to fail to examine a patient who has complained of severe abdominal pain, but it is not negligent to fail to make a diagnosis if an examination is performed and there is no evidence to suggest that under the same circumstances other reasonably skilful doctors would have invariably made the correct diagnosis.

Patients sometimes complain that doctors have been negligent because they have failed to perform all possible tests and examinations. It has to be remembered, however, that in daily practice doctors inevitably take short cuts. If all patients with chest pains were subjected to coronary angiography, for example, there would be little time left for treating patients, the cost would bankrupt the health service and many patients would be put at risk unnecessarily. The fact that doctors do not perform such complex and risky tests on all patients with chest pains inevitably means that some patients with heart disease will not be diagnosed at as early a stage as might have been possible. Nevertheless, the failure to do such a test does not imply negligence. (In America, where patients expect many more tests to be done whether or not they are strictly necessary in medical terms, the situation is rather different.)

Going to the General Medical Council

Set up in 1858 to protect qualified doctors from competition offered by unqualified 'quacks', and to protect the public from the hazards of being treated by incompetent practitioners, the General Medical Council today consists largely of a mixture of nearly a hundred appointed and elected medical practitioners. It is usually regarded as the disciplinary body that twice a year provides the Sunday newspapers with salacious stories about general practitioners accused of sexual misdemeanours by innocent and virginal maidens.

It is sometimes not quite clear from the reports whether a complaint is brought on these occasions because the practitioner did something he should not have done or because he stopped doing something that he should never have started.

Needless to say the General Medical Council does not spend its entire annual budget of nearly £2 million on organizing these public launderings of professional linen. Indeed, most of the cases brought before the General Medical Council's Professional Conduct Committee (until October 1980 known as the Disciplinary Committee) do not involve fornication, adultery, indecent exposure or any other sexual or quasi-sexual activities. Before describing exactly what sort of cases the Professional Conduct Committee is concerned with I'll explain how complaints are usually received.

Responsibilities of the GMC

It is, of course, important to understand that, although the General Medical Council includes among its responsibilities those of maintaining the Medical Register and keeping a check on educational standards in medical schools around the world, it is not concerned with the clinical skills of individual doctors in particular circumstances, unless there is any suggestion that the doctor concerned has failed to fulfil his responsibilities to the patient. In other words if a doctor is asked to visit and he refuses to turn out because it is raining he may be in trouble with the GMC. If, however, he turns out and examines the patient but fails to realize that the patient is suffering from Tibble's disease a complaint is extremely unlikely to merit any sort of investigation.

What happens to a complaint

A complaint sent to the General Medical Council (address on p. 168) will first be studied by a member of the Council's permanent staff who will, with the aid of the GMC President, decide whether or not the complaint deserves any sort of investigation. If the complaint is obviously frivolous then nothing more will happen. If, however, it seems possible that there may be some justification for the complaint then a member of the GMC staff may write to the doctor concerned and ask for his observations. The doctor will not be told the source of the complaint.

The next step is for the GMC staff, under the guidance of the President, to decide whether or not the case should be referred to the Preliminary Proceedings Committee (until October 1980 called the Penal Cases Committee). If it seems likely that there has been some breach of professional discipline (and although the GMC now publishes a booklet entitled *Professional Conduct and Discipline* it refuses to give opinions on whether or not particular actions are likely to result in a case being brought), the Preliminary Proceedings Committee will investigate further.

If the Preliminary Proceedings Committee decides that there is insufficient evidence to warrant the complaint or if it feels that the complaint does not concern the GMC the case will go no further. If the Committee feels that there has been a breach of professional discipline, but that the breach has been a fairly minor one and not one of a long series, then it may send a warning letter to the doctor concerned. If, however, it seems that the complaint is a serious and justified one it will be passed on to the Professional Conduct Committee.

In 1979 the Penal Cases Committee, as it was then called, met three times and considered 99 cases. It referred 30 cases to the Disciplinary Committee (now the Professional Conduct Committee); in 54 cases a warning letter was sent; in 11 cases the complaint was dismissed. The remaining 4 cases were adjourned. At the time that these complaints were made there were 110,806 doctors included on the Medical Register. The 99 cases considered by the Penal Cases Committee were taken out of a total of 920 letters, some of which merely sought advice.

In 1979 the then Disciplinary Committee met three times for a total of 15 days to discuss its 30 cases. One case was withdrawn, one postponed and one abandoned when the doctor applied for voluntary erasure. However, these deletions were more than balanced by the 17 cases brought forward from the previous year either because judgment had been postponed or because a period of temporary suspension had been ordered.

Of the 44 cases actually considered the Disciplinary Committee chose to erase seven doctor's names from the register, to suspend seven temporarily, to postpone judgment in thirteen, to admonish seven and to postpone eight. Two practitioners were found not guilty.

So much for the mechanics of a complaint to the General Medical Council.

The sort of complaint dealt with by the GMC

The type of behaviour which merits a complaint is perhaps of greater interest to the dissatisfied patient.

The first point to make is perhaps rather surprising: today most of the major complaints made to the General Medical Council do not come from patients or even from other doctors but from the courts. Indeed the majority of the complaints heard by both the Penal Cases Committee and the Disciplinary Committee in 1979 came from law court officers; more than 50 per cent of all these complaints involved dishonesty or the abuse of alcohol. After these two major causes of complaints, the third most likely reason for a doctor to find himself before the GMC is the abuse of drugs, and the fourth most likely reason is advertising or canvassing for patients. Even providing patients with false certificates produced more serious complaints than all types of sexual encounters. Over the last few years, the more relaxed legal attitudes towards abortion have meant that it is relatively rare today for any practitioner to find himself before the GMC on a charge of providing a woman with an illegal abortion.

These changes in the type of cases brought before the GMC reflect a change in social attitudes both within and without the medical profession. Today it is by no means certain that a practitioner accused of fornicating with a patient will be struck off the register or even suspended temporarily.

Reasons for complaining about GPs

1 The doctor who has made a mistake or who has failed to provide a patient with proper medical care may make the same mistake again if he is not made aware of his error. It is therefore in the interests of other patients for a complaint to be made.

2 If the error has caused undue suffering or loss of earnings the patient may be entitled to compensation.

3 Doctors are human (although some may not believe this) and are just as likely as other beings to develop mental disorders and other serious problems. Sometimes it is only when a complaint is made that the problems are recognized.

4 The doctor who has taken advantage of a patient's weakened mental or physical condition to further his own economic, social or sexual ambitions provides a threat to the collective reputation of his professional colleagues as well as to the patient.

5 A doctor who practices while under the influence of drugs or alcohol is a menace to his patients and his colleagues as well as himself. He needs help.

6 A doctor who charges patients fees to which he is not entitled is dishonest and patients are entitled to expect their doctors to be honest. There are, after all, many opportunities for the dishonest doctor to take advantage of his situation.

Reasons for not complaining about GPs

1 Everyone makes an occasional mistake and the doctor who makes an error is not necessarily inhuman, immoral, un-ethical or stupid. He may have been tired. He may have simply made a mistake. Whereas lawyers are so accustomed to making faulty judgments that they have a complicated appeals procedure which enables all citizens to appeal against judgments made in court, it is unfortunate that few medical decisions are made in circumstances which allow the customer to insist on a second opinion before accepting any decision that may have been made.

2 Patients who complain about doctors in private or in public do nothing to improve the doctor-patient relationship.

Patients are often encouraged to complain by journalists and social workers who then proceed to grumble about the fact that doctor-patient relationships are often unsatisfactory.

3 The more complaints that are made about doctors the more likely doctors are to start giving patients what they think they want rather than what they may need. For example, many patients would like to have antibiotics prescribed more frequently or X-rays done routinely for minor injuries, but it is now known that there are definite risks associated with antibiotics and X-rays. In addition, the cost of practising what is called 'defensive' medicine can be enormous and the resources available to the NHS are finite (see p. 20).

4 In theory, at least, a doctor about whom a complaint is made could sue for libel if the complaint were frivolous, malicious or unjustified.

5 Complaining about a doctor almost inevitably means finding a new doctor to look after you. Even the most forgiving practitioner will find it difficult to forget the trauma associated with an official complaint.

6 The good doctor will already know that he has made a mistake. A complaint will simply make him suffer more and may affect his ability to practise effectively. A bad doctor will probably not bother at all when a complaint is made. He may not even bother to turn up to a Family Practitioner Committee hearing.

⌐ Specialists

Private specialists

The majority of specialists who offer private medical care are those who also have NHS responsibilities. There are, however, a small number of specialists who work only in the private sector. These are mainly centred in London and in particular in Harley Street.

As far as the private patient is concerned it does not really matter whether a specialist is a whole-time private practitioner or a part-time private practitioner, but the advantages, such as they are, undoubtedly lie with the specialist who has health service connections. He will be able to make use of private beds in NHS hospitals; he will have access to all NHS diagnostic facilities; and he may be more likely to know other specialists to whom he can turn if he needs another opinion.

There is no really effective way for a patient to decide whether or not a specialist is competent. In America an enterprising journalist has published a book called *The Best Doctors in the US* but any such attempt in Britain would be valueless because no reputable specialist will see a patient without a letter of referral from a GP.

A good GP will know which local specialists are competent, which have lengthy waiting lists and which have particular interests in specific subjects (for example, one local surgeon may have a particular interest in thyroid operations while another may be particularly interested in work which involves arterial surgery). He will also know how to get hold of specialists who specialize in particularly rare or difficult-to-manage disorders or who offer unusual forms of treatment. The good GP will know, for example, that the British Association of Plastic

Surgeons publishes an up-to-date list of specialist plastic surgeons together with details of where they work and whether they offer work on the NHS or in private clinics.

Specialists within the National Health Service

The hierarchy within a hospital

A patient in hospital will be looked after not by one doctor but by several. Usually the doctor that patients see most is the house officer, either a junior house physician or house surgeon who is a newly qualified practitioner working on a six-month contract. Every newly qualified doctor must work both as a house physician and a house surgeon before becoming fully registered. Only after registration can a doctor practise outside the hospital service.

The house physicians and the house surgeons are, in theory at least, still in training, but in practice they are unlikely to receive much in the way of post-graduate training. Nor are they likely to be supervised all the time. Indeed, it is the house physicians and house surgeons who usually see patients first when they are admitted to hospital and it is invariably their responsibility to examine the patients and record the first set of notes. In teaching hospitals the first examination may be done by a medical student. If a patient needs medical attention in the night it is usually the house officer who is called first.

The next step on the rung upwards for a hospital doctor is a post as a senior house officer (SHO). At this stage in the medical hierarchy specialization begins and there are SHOs in medicine, surgery, anaesthetics, obstetrics, psychiatry and all other major medical specialities.

Above the SHO comes the junior registrar who may in turn be supervised by a senior registrar. Registrars are officially known as junior doctors although some may be in their late 30s or even early 40s, since in some specialities consultant posts are extremely hard to find.

The responsibilities of the junior hospital doctors vary enormously from hospital to hospital and from speciality to speciality. In some hospitals senior house officers will perform surgical operations on their own, and in almost all hospitals surgical registrars perform operations routinely without consultant supervision. This means that a patient admitted under the care of a consultant may not necessarily be operated on by the consultant himself. This is particularly true of emergency work, which is often done without the consultant being in the hospital at all.

Some patients choosing private practice do so because they argue that they want to be operated on by the consultant and not by a junior doctor. In practice, however, registrars are often just as competent as their seniors and indeed may be more able to deal with routine work. Medical dining rooms frequently hum with the gossip about disasters which have occurred when senior consultants have operated on Very Important Patients suffering from simple disorders. In those instances the consultant may be performing an operation that he has not done for years.

Consultant specialists

It is, of course, every hospital doctor's ambition to become a consultant specialist with authority to admit patients to his own beds and power over his own 'firm' of junior doctors. The age at which doctors achieve consultant status varies a great deal with the speciality they choose. It is, for example, very much easier to become a consultant psychiatrist, consultant geriatrician, consultant anaesthetist or consultant radiologist than to become a consultant general surgeon or consultant plastic surgeon. It is a simple matter of supply and demand. The average age at which junior hospital doctors become consultants is currently 38.

There are naturally many advantages in being a consultant. The basic pay is a little higher, and the status both inside and outside hospitals is considerably greater, but there are in addition all the advantages associated with not having a clinical superior

113

and not having to be on duty within the hospital precincts at all times. (Although consultants are liable to be called in from their homes to deal with emergencies it is in fact relatively rare for them to work outside normal daylight hours.)

There are, moreover, three additional ways in which doctors benefit financially by being appointed as consultants.

First, they are able to perform domiciliary visits when invited to do so by local general practitioners. A consultant receives an extra fee from the National Health Service when he visits patients in their own homes and in some specialities (geriatrics for example) the opportunities of earning extra money this way can be considerable.

Second, consultants are able to choose whether they want to work full time for the National Health Service or whether they want to take part-time contracts and also see private patients. Junior hospital doctors are not allowed this option. The part-time consultant (who is theoretically expected to spend nine-elevenths of his time looking after NHS patients) can sometimes make a considerable amount of money by working in the private sector, and in some specialities (surgery, for example) the potential is enormous. The opportunities for consultant geriatricians, psychiatrists and radiologists to work in private practice are limited and this fact is not unrelated to the fact that entry to these specialities is much easier than entry to the surgical specialities.

The third way that a consultant can improve his income is by obtaining a distinction award. Normally a consultant's annual salary will rise steadily according to a series of nine incremental stages. But in addition to their regular salaries about one-third of the 13,000 NHS consultants will receive a special monetary award. Originally the distinction award system was designed to help reward consultants who had in some way provided a better than average service. It was, literally, intended to reward consultants of special distinction, those with unusual skills or exceptional levels of experience, and those taking out-of-the-ordinary responsibilities.

There are four grades of award in all, ranging from an A-plus award down to a C award. A consultant receiving an A-plus award will find his annual salary more or less doubled, while even consultants receiving C awards will be richer by a considerable sum.

These awards are all made secretly and the identities of consultants receiving extra money are kept very quiet. Even the least cynical of all observers suspect that awards are occasionally made to surgeons choosing to practise full time in the NHS, consultants prepared to accept posts in very unpopular parts of the country and those in unpopular specialities such as geriatrics. More cynical observers claim that awards are made according to the 'old boys' rule and point to the fact that officially released statistics show that London consultants generally do less work, have fewer responsibilities and spend less time on NHS patients than their colleagues outside the capital, and yet are more likely to receive distinction awards.

The harsh fact is that since the NHS was formed there have been sharp discrepancies between the availability of consultants in different areas, and the distinction award system has done nothing to improve matters. If you are a London neurologist you probably stand a much greater chance of having a distinction award than if you are a Birmingham geriatrician, although whether the NHS needs neurologists in London more than geriatricians in Birmingham is debatable.

Getting the best out of a specialist

When a specialist sees you in an out-patients clinic he will have already read a referral letter from your own GP and so he will know something about the problem that has taken you there. If you have been admitted to hospital as an emergency then there will still probably be a referral letter for him to see. If you have been admitted without the knowledge of your GP (directly through the casualty department) then by the time the specialist sees you there will probably be a bulging set of medical notes containing the records compiled by the house officer, the senior house officer and possibly even the registrar.

With this background information already available the specialist is likely to jump to conclusions about your illness. If your GP thinks you have gall bladder disease the specialist is likely to be thinking of gall bladder disease when he sees you. If the admitting house officer thinks you have a chest infection the specialist is likely to be more interested in your chest than your abdomen.

So if you have acquired any additional symptoms since your history was taken, tell the specialist when you see him. Write down your problems on a piece of paper if you think you are likely to forget.

Then when he has finished asking you questions and examining you ask him what conclusions he has drawn and what treatment he is planning to instigate. He should tell you this anyway but some specialists have a nasty tendency to forget that the chests and abdomens they examine belong to real people.

If the specialist does not answer your questions, or if you cannot understand what he tells you (and some specialists tend to find communicating difficult), then ask the house officer or one of the other junior hospital doctors to interpret for you.

Any patient who fails to obtain satisfactory treatment from a specialist or who for some good reason has no faith in him should ask his GP for an alternative referral. Some specialists object to the practice of offering their patients a second specialist opinion, but if given an explanation for the discontent most general practitioners will write a second referral letter. Remember that it is rather difficult (and sometimes impossible) to be switched from one consultant to another when you are an in-patient in hospital.

Finally, do remember that while specialists provide technical advice the best person to discuss possible treatment plans with is your own family doctor. When he has received a reply to his original referral letter he will be able to explain exactly what advice the specialist has offered. Together you can then decide whether or not to accept the recommended treatment.

Ethical dilemmas

In general, the ethical problems facing hospital practitioners and patients in hospital are similar to those facing GPs and patients in the community. There are, however, some differences, partly because hospital specialists, unlike GPs, do not have total responsibility for their patients, partly because hospital specialists are employed members of an institutional team, and partly because the diagnostic and therapeutic aids employed in hospitals are considerably more complex in technological terms than the aids employed in general practice.

Regrettably it is true that some hospital specialists seem to regard their patients less as human beings than as breathing pathology specimens. There is certainly plenty of evidence to suggest that some consultants perform tests and investigations regardless of the needs of the individual patient and directly for their own interest. Teaching hospital consultants seem particularly likely to behave in this way.

Other ethical problems which concern hospital practitioners rather than general practitioners include transplantation of organs, psychosurgery, electroconvulsive therapy, the teaching of medical students and the organization of trials involving untried forms of treatment.

Most modern hospitals have ethical committees which are supposed to safeguard the patients and which should, theoretically, provide a check on over-enthusiastic specialists, but whether such committees exist or not it seems to me that the patient's own GP is probably the best person to advise on whether or not a particular investigation or treatment should be tried.

The patient's GP is, after all, the only doctor who is unlikely to have a personal interest in the outcome of any hospital research programme (many hospital doctors openly recognize that career prospects in the hospital service depend upon the number of research papers they have published) and may in addition be the best person to explain any suggested forms of treatment and to interpret any advice, suggestions or recommendations that the patient may have received.

Complaining about a specialist or any other hospital doctor

Legal action

A patient who wishes to complain about the quality of clinical treatment he has received or who wants to institute legal proceedings against a practitioner he suspects of negligence is entitled to take the appropriate action through the law courts. The type of action which is usually described as 'negligence' is described on p. 104, in the section dealing with complaints about general practitioners.

It is perhaps worth pointing out here that there is now undisputed evidence that the growing rate at which patients take legal action against doctors has undoubtedly led to many changes in clinical attitudes in recent years. For example, it seems possible that the increase in the number of obstetricians opting to deliver babies by Cesarian section may be linked to a well publicized legal case which involved a consultant obstetrician accused of handing his forceps negligently. The surgeon eventually won his case but to do so he had to fight through the law courts for a number of years. It is perhaps not surprising that other doctors should try to avoid similar situations by allowing legal rather than clinical considerations to colour their attitudes.

A complaint to the GMC

It is, of course, also possible for a patient, relative or anyone else to make a complaint to the General Medical Council if it is felt that any practitioner has behaved in an unprofessional manner. Again the rules which relate to complaints to the GMC are the same as the ones relating to complaints about general practitioners. These are outlined on pp. 105–108.

The majority of complaints about hospital doctors do not, however, warrant or justify legal proceedings or complaints to the General Medical Council and there is a special complaints procedure in operation designed to deal with the sort of complaints that would be referred to the Family Practitioner Committee if they involved a general practitioner.

A complaint to the hospital

The simplest and most straightforward way to institute a complaint is to approach the head of the department concerned or the senior hospital administrator. Like workers in all branches of the NHS, hospital staff of all grades are particularly sensitive to criticism and will usually consider even the flimsiest complaint very carefully indeed.

Once the local administrator or the consultant in charge of the department concerned has made his investigation a report should be sent to the complainant either offering an explanation or an apology. If no such report is forthcoming or if the complainant is not satisfied with the response he gets he is perfectly entitled to take his complaint a stage higher, writing either to the District Management Team or the Regional Health Authority. (A full account of the way in which the NHS is constructed appears on pp. 17–20.)

A patient or a relative of a patient or a representative of a patient who has a complaint of any kind (whether or not it involves a medical practitioner) is entitled to make a complaint in this way. A complaint about hospital porters, about hospital food, about visiting times, about car parking facilities or about anything else, can be made in exactly the same way as a complaint about the activities of hospital doctors.

Other ways to complain

In addition to these avenues for complaint there are two other routes that complainants can follow.

First, anyone who has a complaint about treatment and who wants more information is now entitled to a meeting with the doctors concerned and to a written explanation. If the explanation that comes from the relevant doctors is not satisfactory then the Regional Medical Officer (a full-time medical administrator) can be brought into the dispute. If his explanation still does not provide the patient with a satisfactory account of what has happened there is a third stage: the complainant can have his problem considered by two consultants from an entirely different area.

The other route that can be followed is designed to cope with complaints about administrative organization or about non-clinical aspects of hospital care. Should the complainant have had his allegation considered by the local administrator and still have failed to obtain a satisfactory response he is entitled to make a complaint to the Health Service Commissioner, otherwise known as the NHS Ombudsman.

The Health Service Commissioner is responsible directly to Parliament, not to the DHSS, and has the power to investigate any allegation that involves a charge of maladministration and has already been investigated by the Health Authority concerned. He is not allowed to investigate charges of clinical negligence and he will not reopen a case if he is satisfied that it has been investigated properly at a local level.

The Health Service Commissioner's post and responsibilities are modelled on those of the Parliamentary Commissioner for Administration (also known as the Ombudsman) who was originally given power to deal with maladministration by civil servants (Richard Crossman described the Ombudsman's duties as involving cases of 'neglect, inattention, delay, incompetence, ineptitude, perversity, turpitude and so on'), but whose brief is basically to question the way in which decisions have been reached rather than the nature of these decisions. It is an important part of the Health Services Commissioner's role to see that local health service officials have dealt efficiently and compassionately with any complaints that have been made.

The local Community Health Council

It will be clear from what I have written so far that making a complaint about any part of the hospital service is a complicated business and it may help to recruit the help and professional advice of the Secretary to the local Community Health Council who can usually be reached via the local telephone directory. If you have difficulty in obtaining the relevant address try the local Family Practitioner Committee, any local hospital administrator or the reference section of the local library. Should there be no Community Health Council Secretary available then preliminary advice about how to make a complaint can be obtained through the Health Service Commissioner at Church House, Great Smith Street, London SW1P 3BW.

It is obviously wise to make any complaint as soon as possible since memories fade and records may disappear as time passes.

A to Z directory of specialists

anaesthetist
Uses drugs, sometimes given by injection and sometimes administered as gases, to send patients to sleep, usually so that surgeons can then operate on them. Anaesthetists also specialize in using drugs to relieve pain and in many hospitals they are also given the responsibility of looking after patients who are for any reason unconscious.

cardiologist
A physician who deals exclusively with disorders of the heart. Most patients who have heart attacks will be looked after by general physicians, but rare or difficult to treat cardiac conditions may merit a second referral to a cardiologist. In large centres where there is a resident cardiologist all patients with heart conditions may be referred.

child psychiatrist
A psychiatrist who has chosen to specialize in the mental problems of children. Difficult, withdrawn or over-active children may all be referred to a child psychiatrist.

clinical physiologist
Specializes in relating the way in which the body works (or does not work) to specific disease processes. Although he deals with real patients (as opposed to theories and animals) the clinical physiologist is still often something of a back room boy.

community health physician
Theoretically responsible for supervising the provision of health care within the community, but in practice more often a member of the NHS administration who has little contact with patients.

dermatologist
Specializes in skin problems of all kinds. Although family doctors deal with the vast majority of rashes and skin ailments dermatologists are often called in to help with the treatment of persistent problems. Sufferers of bad acne, eczema and psoriasis may see a dermatologist.

ear, nose and throat surgeon
Usually known as an ENT specialist. The tonsillectomy is the most common operation performed by ENT surgeons. Sinus problems and hearing problems may also merit referral to the ENT specialist.

endocrinologist
A physician who deals exclusively with problems associated with the hormone-producing glands within the body. There are relatively few endocrinologists in Britain and most of them work in major centres. Endocrinologists usually deal with such

problems as deficiencies of growth hormone rather than with disorders associated with the thyroid gland or pancreas gland (see p. 268).

forensic pathologist
Specializes in studying the bodies of those who have been victims of violence but also takes a general interest in the areas where medicine and the law overlap. Patients are unlikely ever to know anything about a referral to a forensic pathologist.

forensic psychiatrist
Deals exclusively with mentally ill patients who have committed crimes or who are suspected of having committed crimes.

gastroenterologist
Specialist physician who deals with problems affecting the intestines. Like many physicians specializing in particular areas of medicine he may also see patients with problems outside his own speciality. For example, a gastroenterologist may also have patients with rheumatism or heart disease referred to him. There are, however, some gastroenterologists (usually working in large or teaching hospitals) who deal *only* with problems such as ulcerative colitis, Crohn's disease and so on.

geriatrician
Deals only with the elderly – usually people over the age of sixty-five. Some doctors argue that there is no real justification for a speciality dealing with the elderly since people over sixty-five suffer from very much the same range of disorders as younger patients. However, the number of hospitals exclusively for patients over sixty-five (or thereabouts) means that there is a need for doctors to specialize.

gynaecologist
Specializes in women's problems and all the disorders which affect females 'down below'. Fibroids, ovarian cysts, unusual bleeding, painful periods and so on are problems often dealt with by gynaecologists. Most gynaecologists are also obstetricians.

haematologist
Deals with problems of the blood. Usually works in a laboratory but does see patients – usually at the request of a specialist physician. Will advise on the treatment of problems such as anaemia and leukaemia.

nephrologist
Deals with problems associated with the kidneys. The nephrologist is, in practice, often more interested in physiology that in anatomical abnormalities, which are usually the province of the urologist. A nephrologist will usually only be consulted when a patient has already been referred to a hospital specialist. Most nephrologists work in special centres.

neuroradiologist
Specializes in taking pictures of the nervous system with the aid of X-rays, scanners and so on.

neurosurgeon
Specialist surgeon who operates on the nervous system, including the brain. Will operate to remove blood clots, brain tumours, etc. Usually found only in specialist centres.

obstetrician
Looks after pregnant women before, during and after delivery. Is often also a gynaecologist.

occupational health specialist
Physician who deals with the disorders associated with particular types of employment. Many large companies employ their own occupational health specialist to help prevent disease and to help deal with employees who have contracted disorders at work.

oncologist
Doctor who specializes in the diagnosis and treatment of cancer. Most patients with cancer will be looked after by other specialists, but occasionally one of the few oncologists in the country will be called in if there is a rare disorder to treat or an unusual remedy to try.

ophthalmologist
An eye specialist. Deals with problems such as cataracts, glaucoma, retinal detachment and severe eye infections.

orthopaedic surgeon
Specializes in bones and joints and the various problems which can afflict these structures. Orthopaedic surgeons deal with slipped discs, arthritis and cartilage problems, and with fractures of all kinds. Because there is a steady demand for the services of orthopaedic surgeons from accident victims, patients awaiting routine surgery (e.g. hip replacement surgery) may have to wait a long time. Waiting lists tend to be very long in orthopaedics, but can often be cut dramatically if private treatment is sought since orthopaedic surgeons have to deal with few emergencies in their private practice. Casualty departments are often run by orthopaedic surgeons.

paediatrician
Specialist in the care of children who will deal with *all* the ailments affecting children. The age at which a child will be passed on to an ordinary specialist varies according to the child, and the paediatrician, and the illness.

pathologist
Dissects dead bodies, examines biopsy specimens and supervises work in the pathology laboratory (see p. 191). Unlikely to be seen by live patients.

pharmacologist
An expert in the preparation and use of drugs. May or may not be seen by patients. May or may not be clinically qualified. Usually a back room boy (or girl).

physician
Someone who deals exclusively with medical, rather than surgical, problems. General physicians sometimes have their favourite specialities (diabetes, gastroenterology, liver problems, etc.). Whatever other specialists there may be, most hospitals will have at least one general physician and one general surgeon.

plastic surgeon
Performs operations designed to improve the function and appearance of the human body. It is true that some plastic surgeons (usually known as cosmetic surgeons) spend all their time making small breasts larger and large breasts smaller but others do a considerable amount of work on burn and accident victims. The demand for the services offered by plastic surgeons far exceeds the supply and waiting lists for 'cosmetic' operations are often very long within the health service.

proctologist
A doctor who specializes in the lower end of the intestinal tract. Piles are not the beginning and end of a proctologist's work but they make up quite a proportion of it.

psychiatrist
Will deal exclusively with mental problems. Psychiatrists are called in by both GPs and hospital specialists where patients seem to need psychiatric help. Psychiatrists deal with individuals suffering from short-term problems such as mild depression and with individuals suffering from severe, long-term problems such as schizophrenia.

psychotherapist
Specializes in providing support for those with mental problems, usually on an individual, one-to-one basis. Not all psychotherapists are medically qualified; the time required for treatment means that the availability of psychotherapy within the NHS is severely limited.

radiologist
Supervises the taking of X-rays (by a radiographer) and reads the resultant plates before making a written report for the benefit of the patient's physician.

radiotherapist
Someone who uses ray treatment (see p. 302) to help patients. Many of the radiotherapist's patients are cancer sufferers.

rheumatologist
Physician who specializes in the treatment of rheumatic disorders such as rheumatoid arthritis, osteoarthritis, gout and so on.

surgeon
Someone whose skills are applied with the knife rather than the stethoscope. A general surgeon will operate on just about anyone to remove just about anything or to repair any fault. Some surgeons specialize in, for example, brain surgery, heart surgery etc.

thoracic surgeon
Specialist surgeon who operates on the chest and does surgical operations on the lungs and heart. Sometimes known affectionately as a 'chest cutter'.

urologist
Specializes in problems involving the bladder, kidneys and other parts of the urinary system.

venereologist
Specializes in diagnosing and treating diseases of the sexual organs. That usually means diseases, such as syphilis, transmitted by sexual intercourse.

Other Professionals

A to Z directory of other professionals

A century ago when medicine was a relatively simple business and doctors could do relatively little to ease discomfort or disrupt disease processes there were few, if any, supplementary medical professions. Today, as progress continues annually, the need for technical specialists increases regularly. Within the medical profession specialists begin to find a need to specialize in one branch of their chosen subject; outside the profession there is a growing demand for specialists able to deal with specific problems or to operate specific pieces of machinery. This need does not simply arise from the fact that doctors are too busy to do everything – the truth is that doctors are no longer able to master all the technical equipment and the specific skills which the profession has introduced. The addresses for the relevant professional organizations can be found in the directory beginning on p. 166.

chiropodists
To be recognized as qualified by the Society of Chiropodists and by the Chiropodists Board of the Council for Professions Supplementary to Medicine, chiropodists must spend three years on full-time study and become state registered. To work within the health service a chiropodist must be state registered and no specialist without this qualification should, in my opinion, be consulted. In some circumstances GPs will refer patients to chiropodists. However, chiropodists can be seen without a referral. Local telephone directories usually carry names and addresses.

dentists
Qualified dentists register with the General Dental Council whether they practise privately or solely within the health service. Most dentists in general practice do some health service and some private work. No dentist is obliged to take health service patients, and it seems that relatively few do complicated work on anyone other than private patients. The yellow pages of the telephone directory contain a list of dentists and the local Family Practitioner Committee will also be able to provide a list. Dentists do not have to provide any emergency cover; they do not have to see patients a second time just because they have seen them once; and they are not paid to provide any advice about prevention of dental decay. In fact, since they are paid only for looking after bad teeth the dental profession does have a vested interest in ensuring that dental hygiene in Britain remains poor. Fortunately, most dentists are too conscientious to allow such mercenary thoughts to enter their minds.

Dentists are allowed to provide check-ups, mend false teeth and arrest haemorrhages without making any charge. Fillings, extractions and cleaning of the teeth are paid for partly by the health service and partly by the patient. A patient who needs false teeth or more complicated work will have to pay the agreed health service cost. Children, pregnant women, people receiving free prescriptions, people receiving supplementary benefit or family income supplements, and some students, will be entitled to free treatment, but the dentist must be told at the time of the treatment, and a form must be signed.

Dental therapists and dental hygienists work under the supervision of dentists and provide a number of the simpler services. Dental nurses do not usually need any official training. Their job is to assist the dentist and distract the patient.

Complaints about dental care should be made to the local Family Practitioner Committee if the complaint concerns the standard of care or the service provided and to the General Dental Council if the complaint concerns the dentist's personal or ethical behaviour.

dieticians

A great many diseases and disorders can be made worse by eating the wrong foods and made better by eating the right amounts of the right foods. Peptic ulcers, diabetes, gall bladder trouble, heart disease and colitis are just a few of the disorders directly linked to diet. Knowing which foods can be of benefit to which patients is a complex job and trained and qualified dieticians play an important part in medical care. Most of them work in hospitals where they provide daily advice for the catering staffs. Inevitably dieticians spend a good deal of time working with the overweight and many have printed literature and sample diets available for patients. In some areas GPs can refer their patients directly to a local hospital dietician.

home helps

Home helps come under the authority of the local social services department. In my view they provide the most important part of the service provided by that department. It is the job of the home help to help with all the household tasks that the 'client' finds too difficult — cleaning, shopping, cooking and so on are the main tasks involved. Most home helps are allocated to help the elderly, who would otherwise find it impossible to live at home, and the time they spend with each individual or each couple varies from a few hours to a few days a week. A charge is made for a home help according to the resources of the individual who is being helped. GPs have no control over the allocation of home helps, but may be able to help applicants with a note of support. Applications should be made to the Director of Social Services in the area concerned.

Home helps are not expected to have any qualifications: the most important requirements are patience and enthusiasm.

medical laboratory technicians

Even quite small hospitals have to deal with and test a large number of personal samples every day. There are blood and urine samples, of course, but in addition there are swabs of discharges and infective growths to be examined, and faecal samples to be studied. Complex machinery sometimes enables technicians to test many samples at once and to assess a number of different values in one examination.

nurses

Nurses are, of course, vitally important to all branches of medical care and no medical institution could operate effectively without them. Many of the hospitals throughout

Britain run nursing schools where students can enrol either to follow a course of practical and theoretical studies leading to the qualification of state registration (entitling the holder to use the letters SRN after his or her name) or to follow an academically slightly less arduous course leading to the qualification of state enrolment (which entitles the holder to use the letters SEN after his or her name). These two qualifications, SRN and SEN, are the two fundamental, basic qualifications, without which no nurse can claim to be a real professional.

In addition to being state registered or enrolled nurses can gather a specialist qualification. The General Nursing Council recognizes a number of other courses and examinations and nurses who have followed the appropriate course of training and passed the necessary examination will be entitled to add different letters after their names. A registered mental nurse will be described as RMN, a registered nurse of the mentally subnormal will be RMNS; a state enrolled nurse who has specialized in the care of the mentally ill or the mentally subnormal will have the letters SEN(M) or SEN(MS) after his or her name. A registered nurse tutor is entitled to the letters RNT while a registered clinical nurse teacher is entitled to the letters RCNT. A registered sick children's nurse uses the letters RSCN.

Nurses who have specialized in the care of sick children or the mentally ill will, of course, usually work in the appropriate hospitals. General nurses may work either in hospitals or in the community. Within the hospital environment there is a strict hierarchy for nurses with the newly qualified staff nurse being on the bottom rung of the professional career structure, the junior sister (or in the case of a male nurse, charge nurse) being on the next rung up and an apparently unending series of administrative nurses occupying more senior posts. State enrolled nurses are not entitled to rise within the nursing structure.

In the community both state enrolled and state registered nurses can work 'on the district' although the range of work that a registered nurse can do is rather wider than the range that is within the province of a state enrolled nurse (see p. 50). As in hospitals there is an extensive career structure in community care for nurses although the more senior nursing officers rarely come into contact with patients.

midwives

Nurses who wish to practise midwifery (see p. 57) must follow an additional course and as with general nurses there are openings for qualified and registered midwives both within hospitals, where they will work in maternity units, or in the community where they will arrange ante- and post-natal classes in addition to looking after a limited number of births at home.

health visitors

There are a number of nurses working as health visitors. A nursing qualification (as a state registered nurse) is an essential prerequisite but a further period of training leads to additional certification. Health visitors are expected to spend time looking after the very young and the very old and are, in theory at least, expected to offer advice about the prevention of disease (see also p. 57).

Any properly qualified nurse who fails to satisfy accepted professional standards can be disciplined by the General Nursing Council.

occupational therapists

Looking after the patient's mind is often as important as looking after his body and this is particularly true during a long illness or during a period of convalescence. Patients who are confined to bed or who are temporarily or permanently disabled in some way may not be able to follow their usual occupation or hobby and it is the job of the occupational therapist to suggest and provide alternatives, either in an attempt to find a solution to temporary boredom or in an attempt to find a solution to what might otherwise be permanent unemployment. Occupational therapy has in recent years become a considered science and practitioners today spend a considerable amount of time and energy searching for ways to capture the imagination of their patients and to encourage physical and mental rehabilitation.

opticians

There are, in Britain, two types of opticians. Ophthalmic opticians who test sight also supply and fit optical appliances (that is the term used by the General Optical Council), while dispensing opticians do not test sight but will supply and fit optical appliances. Ophthalmic surgeons are qualified doctors who have specialized in the study of eye disorders and who are entitled to treat eye problems with medicines, surgery or spectacles as they see fit. You can simply walk into any suitable optician if you want to have your eyes tested. The test can be done free on the NHS and you do not need a letter from your GP. There is a fixed charge payable for health service lenses and frames but more fashionable frames have to be paid for privately. Some individuals (for example, those receiving family income supplement) can obtain basic spectacles without charge.

orthoptists

Orthoptists are specialists in orthoptics which is the treatment of squints by exercising the eye muscles.

physiotherapists

Physiotherapy simply means physical therapy but today's physiotherapists have turned those two simple words into a real science. With the aid of both simple gymnasium equipment and complex electrical equipment they can often work wonders in helping partly paralysed stroke and accident victims to regain their strength. They can also help asthmatic and bronchitic patients by teaching them ways to improve breathing and expel phlegm.

remedial gymnasts

Whereas physiotherapy involves passive as well as active movements (in other words the physiotherapist may provide the power) remedial gymnasts help patients by teaching them to exercise and encouraging them to use their own muscles.

school health officials

Britain's school health clinics are run by doctors, dentists and nurses. The aim is to ensure that outbreaks of infectious disease are avoided (this is difficult to do in view of the irregularity and infrequency of the inspections); to spot signs of physical or mental abnormality; and to offer advice where appropriate. The school dental service, unlike the school medical services, is both a diagnostic and a treatment service. Whereas doctors in the school clinics do not provide any sort of treatment (they usually refer patients back to their GP or, with his approval, directly to a hospital specialist) dentists do carry out suitable forms of treatment.

social workers

The Department of Health and Social Security is represented in the government by the Secretary of State for Social Services, who is responsible for (1) the health services, which provide all forms of medical care, (2) the social security system, which provides financial support for the elderly, the disabled and the ill, and others in financial need, and (3) Personal Social Services, which provide supporting care within the community for all those in need of non-medical help.

Although the DHSS in London provides some advice and some money, social services are organized by all the major local authorities which must appoint social services committees and departments. Each committee and therefore each department is expected to provide services designed to help in the care of the elderly, the homeless and the physically handicapped, children needing residential accommodation, and the mentally disordered needing support. It is the local social services committee which is expected to provide home helps, to supervise day nurseries and the licensing of child minders, to provide care for unsupported mothers and to keep a number of trained social workers available to help individuals in need.

Social services departments vary from authority to authority but most have a headquarters which includes staff detailed to look after residential services, community care, and training. Incidentally, social workers, who love jargon even more than doctors do, usually describe community care as field work services. In addition to a headquarters staff, there will usually be area or district teams consisting of a number of social workers expected to look after the people living in that area. A second important piece of jargon is the word 'client' which is always used by social workers to describe the individuals seeking their help.

Social workers undoubtedly provide a number of people with an important service and they organize and operate a variety of essential facilities. It is unfortunate that they have in recent years acquired a public reputation for caring more about paperwork, committees and status than about the clients for whom they are theoretically responsible. Sadly the career structure within the social services is such that only relatively junior workers have any real face to face contact with ordinary citizens. Most social workers do not have technical or academic qualifications but a growing number have degrees or diplomas in social studies or social sciences.

others

There is a growing number of other professionals involved in health care. Audiology technicians operate the equipment used to test hearing. ECG technicians operate the equipment used to study the human heart and EEG technicians operate the equipment used to study brain waves. Speech therapists specialize in helping individuals who have difficulty in speaking and they spend time with patients of all ages. There are training programmes designed to teach would-be nursery nurses the basic facts about the care of infants and young children.

Private nurses

The shortage of suitable nursing home accommodation, the cost of such accommodation when it can be found, and the reluctance of both the invalid concerned and his or her relatives to consider institutional accommodation as a realistic alternative to home care mean that in many cases the frail, the convalescent and the elderly must remain in the care of relatives and friends who may not have the time, the equipment or the training to provide the type of attention required.

The district nursing service provided by local authorities and usually coordinated by GPs can do a great deal to help but there are severe limitations on the extent of the care available through this public service. These statutory facilities can, however, be supplemented by the use of private nurses.

There are a number of nursing associations and organizations in Britain offering the services of private nurses but the largest commercial agency is the British Nursing Association which acts as an introduction agency for nurses all over Britain. The BNA has 40 branches which operate 24 hours a day for seven days a week, and offers only qualified nurses. The cost of hiring a nurse, either on a full-time or part-time basis, is not inconsiderable but the advantages of home care may be great. Some private insurance schemes cover the cost of private nursing care and home attendance allowances may help towards the cost (see p. 316). The address of the British Nursing Association's head office (from which details of the provincial agencies can be obtained) is 470 Oxford Street, London W1N 0HQ. Other organizations which may be of use can be found listed on pp. 174 ff.

Under the Nurses Agencies Act of 1957 it is illegal to run a nurses' agency without a licence.

Alternative Professionals

Why people use alternative medicine and why they should take care when they do

The number and variety of alternative or fringe forms of medical treatment rise each year. One important reason is undoubtedly the fact that an increasing number of people are becoming disillusioned and unhappy with orthodox or allopathic medicine. They are unhappy because the barriers which separate patients and doctors seem to grow annually, because the availability of professional medical care seems to decline in direct proportion to the demand, and because of the growing disenchantment with the medical establishment fired by the failure of allopathic practitioners to recognize and effectively halt the rising incidence of side effects related to the use of modern forms of investigation and treatment.

Unhappily, although the problems may be different there are undoubtedly as many difficulties associated with unorthodox medical treatments as there are with the orthodox, establishment practices. To begin with it is important for all consumers to recognize that alternative forms of medicine are not automatically devoid of risk. The dangers may be different from the dangers associated with surgery or drug therapy but they are without doubt just as real. And although it is certainly true that the better qualified, more experienced, more cautious and less dramatic practitioners are certainly safer than those who are less experienced and more flamboyant, the consumer has no way of differentiating between the good and the terrible in the world of alternative medicine. A truly incompetent medical practitioner will lose his licence to practice. A truly incompetent unorthodox practitioner cannot be banned or removed from any register because the chances are high that he was not on any official list to begin with. His unfortunate patients may have an

133

additional disadvantage; since their practitioner is unlikely to be insured for the consequences of negligence, they may find that he is without the means to satisfy any judgment they may get for the damage done.

A to Z guide to alternative medicine

On the following pages I have tried to provide a brief introductory account of some of the commoner forms of unorthodox medicine. I suspect that some of my critical comments may not please those who practise within these various disciplines. I excuse myself on two grounds: first, I have been equally critical of orthodox medical practices that I consider worthy of criticism; second, it seems to me to be unreasonable to insist that medical practitioners and pharmaceutical companies provide proof of the efficacy of their activities without insisting that similar conditions be met by unorthodox practitioners. I suggest that readers who would like to study more thoroughly the history and application of 'alternative' forms of medicine read *Natural Medicine* by Brian Inglis, published by Collins in 1979.

Incidentally, practitioners in these various disciplines are not restricted or governed by any specific legislation. Although I have listed at the end of this section a selection of some of the 'qualifications' awarded to practitioners there is no simple way for patients to judge the quality or reliability of an individual practitioner. My inclusion of these qualifications does not in any way imply that I recommend those individuals possessing the qualifications. It is also important to remember that 'fringe' practitioners are not authorized to sign official certificates (such as death certificates, health service prescriptions and so on) and although many of them do sign sick notes there is no legal obligation on any agency to accept or acknowledge the notes.

acupuncture

Imported from China, this technique involves the use of many small needles usually made of pure silver or gold. These needles are pushed into the skin and although the treatment sounds terribly painful skilled practitioners insist that it is not. The needles are inserted in such a way as to influence the central nervous system and have an effect on whichever part of the body is out of balance. Researchers have attempted to explain just how and why acupuncture works but have so far failed to come up with any solid scientific explanation. Nevertheless, the technique has undoubtedly been used with great effect particularly in the treatment of pain and to provide anaesthesia. The main problem facing the consumer is in finding a reliable practitioner. If the acupuncturist does not sterilize his needles properly there is a real risk of infection and hepatitis outbreaks have been caused by badly cleaned needles. There is as yet no register of acupuncturists in the same way that there is a Register of Medical Practitioners but reliable practitioners can usually be found either through a helpful general practitioner (who will know which local acupuncturist to recommend) or through the British Acupuncture Association (see p. 167).

Alexander Method, Principle or Technique

Named after Frederick Matthias Alexander who died in London in 1955, this form of treatment is said to be an effective remedy for stress. It involves training the body's muscles and controlling the tension within them. Effectively a form of relaxation therapy the Alexander Method can probably be studied best through one of the many books on the subject.

baths and bathing

Cold baths, hot baths, saunas, turkish baths, salt baths, foam baths, alternating baths, foot baths, sitzbaths, jet baths, whirlpools, steam baths – and on the list goes. All these forms of treatment can be pooled together under the generic term 'hydrotherapy' and although they may make those who enjoy them feel relaxed, clean and fresh they are unlikely to have any genuine medicinal qualities.

biochemistry

The form of treatment usually described under this heading has nothing to do with the branch of science which bears the same name. In purely scientific terms biochemistry is defined as the science of living matter. As a form of treatment, however, the word is used to describe the system devised by Dr Wilhelm Schussler who showed that when in good health every human body includes quantities of each of twelve salts (calcium fluoride, calcium phosphate, calcium sulphate, ferrous phosphate, potassium chloride, potassium phosphate, potassium sulphate, sodium chloride, sodium phosphate, sodium sulphate, magnesium phosphate, and silicic oxide). He claimed that one or more of these salts was missing from the body in any illness and that the treatment of an illness simply involved replacing the missing salts. To the best of my knowledge there is absolutely no indisputable scientific evidence supporting this theory.

biofeedback

Biofeedback relies on the patient learning how to assess and control normal physiological responses. For example, the patient is taught to be aware of his or her own heartbeat and to control the beat voluntarily.
Suggested reading: *Biofeedback: Turning on the Power of Your Mind* by Marvin Karlins and Lewis M. Andrews. Published by Abacus, 1975.

chiropractic

Basically chiropractors offer their patients a type of manipulation. Benefits can undoubtedly be obtained when the aim is to treat muscular or bone problems. Some chiropractors claim to be able to treat a much wider range of disorders but I know of no evidence for their claims. There is in practice little or no difference between chiropractic and osteopathy although I suspect that members of both disciplines would hotly dispute that statement.

diatetics

Very many different disciplines and philosophies fall within this simple category but most of them involve the use of particular minerals or vitamins or the exclusion of specific foodstuffs from the diet. Since it is more difficult to make money by telling people what not to eat than by telling them what to eat, most diatetic experts who campaign publicly advocate the addition of some specific product to the diet. I have described the importance of vitamins elsewhere in this book (see p. 279) but my brief comment is that anyone who eats a good, balanced diet does not need and will not benefit from any additional minerals, vitamins or other foodstuffs.

gravitonics

Although it is said to be quite popular in America this form of therapy has not caught on in Britain. The proponents suggest that followers erect trapeze-like structures between their doorposts and spend part of the day hanging upside down. This is said to be good for physical strains and emotional hang-ups.

herbalism

Followers of herbalism claim that the use of plants for their medicinal qualities is safer and more natural than the use of chemicals. They forget, of course, that many drugs used by traditional practitioners (or allopathic doctors) either consist of or are based on herbal extracts. Many herbal remedies undoubtedly work but there are risks and dangers associated with this form of treatment and plant extracts need to be treated with respect. Morphine, digitalis and aspirin were originally obtained from plants and trees.

Suggested reading: *Healing Plants* by William A. R. Thompson. Published by Macmillan, 1980.

holistic medicine

Many doctors have in recent years been accused of treating diseases rather than people and of being interested in organs rather than patients. Aware of the justifications for this accusation a number of modern doctors are now practising holistic medicine. This simply means that they regard all forms of therapy as potentially worthwhile (whether they are accepted by the stricter traditionalists or not) and they consider that their aim is to treat the patient, not the disease or an isolated part of the body.

homoeopathy

Founded by the German, Samuel Hahnemann, this form of treatment has strong links with orthodox, allopathic medicine. Minute doses of drugs are given with the intention of triggering a defensive reaction within the body and stimulating the body's own natural resistance to disease, much in the same way that doctors use vaccine and drinkers take 'a hair of the dog'. The homoeopathic practitioner will prescribe a drug which would, if given in larger doses, produce the very symptoms of which his patient complains. For example, he will give a very nervous patient a minute dose of coffee because in larger doses coffee causes a greater sense of nervous awareness. To prepare their medicines homoeopathic practitioners effectively empty a bottle of neat medicine into a lake and then use the lake water as medicine. Because of the fact that medicines are given in such a diluted form, side effects and bad reactions are relatively rare in homoeopathy.

Suggested reading: *Homoeopathy, An Introductory Guide* by A. C. Gordon Ross. Published by Thorsons, 1979.

hydrotherapy

see baths and bathing.

137

hypnosis

Since it was first introduced by Mesmer in the 18th century hypnosis has had rather a bad press. Part of the problem has undoubtedly been caused by the fact that many 'stage hypnotists' have rather cheapened the art and have encouraged members of the public to associate hypnotism with charlatans, cheats and confidence tricksters. The orthodox medical profession has not been unwilling to support this suspicion. The truth seems to be that although not all individuals are susceptible to hypnotherapy this form of treatment can be extremely effective when used professionally and when its limitations are recognized. It can, for example, be used in the treatment of fears, anxieties and addictions and in the alleviation of physical disorders associated with psychological problems such as bed-wetting, stammering and high blood pressure.

Suggested reading: *Hypnosis, Fact and Fiction* by F. L. Marcuse. Published by Penguin, 1959. *New Hope Through Hypnotherapy* by Monica O'Hara. Published by Abacus, 1980.

meditation

My own feeling about meditation is that the publicity given to the procedure by the more outrageous advocates has discouraged many millions of potential students. The simple truth is that you do not have to shave your head, wear strange robes, sell long-playing records in public places, pay out vast sums of money or join any one of the numerous sects and organizations offering to teach you how to meditate in order to benefit from this undoubtedly useful way of dealing with some of life's problems. There is powerful, convincing evidence that by learning to meditate individuals can not only deal with mental problems and psychological stresses but that they can also control a wide range of associated physical disorders.

Suggested reading: *Stress Control* by Vernon Coleman. Published by Pan Books, 1980.

music therapy

Music was used thousands of years ago in Greece as a form of therapy and during the intervening centuries many individuals have found the right kind of music soothing and calming. To benefit from music therapy all you need is to buy a record player or tape recorder and the appropriate records or tapes.

nature cure

The term 'nature cure' usually refers to the sort of treatment obtainable at health farms and hydros where the paying customers are subjected to conditions that are common in two-thirds of the world — fasting being the most important part of the cure (see pp. 157–58). Exposure to the elements is also considered to be an integral part of many 'nature cures' and there is a growing number of people who believe that the human body should be totally exposed whenever possible. The rise in popularity of nudist camps and nude bathing beaches cannot, however, be entirely explained by the benefits accruing to the health of the individuals concerned.

osteopathy
Founded by Andrew Still who was himself medically qualified, osteopathy is an important, self-supporting branch of medicine. The practitioners who follow Still's example are more than simple bone setters and many can claim with good reason to offer a wide range of medical services. Their most important activities, however, are undoubtedly concerned with the abnormalities associated with the human frame and skilled osteopaths can often deal with dislocations, slipped discs, back pains, and all the various forms of rheumatism and arthritis far more effectively than their allopathic colleagues.

phrenology
This unusual speciality is usually referred to as the reading of bumps on the human head and, like hypnosis, it has suffered from its association with fairs and circuses. Phrenologists, who sometimes call themselves phrenoanalysts, claim to be able to study character and human frailties by examining human heads.

radiesthesia and radionics
Of all the forms of alternative medicine this is probably the one most difficult to describe or assess. In principle radiesthesia is rather similar to water divining – both rely on the fact that the operator is sensitive to vibrations emanating from the source being sought or studied. Radiesthesists around the world have conducted many studies of the vibrations involved but so far I have not seen any orthodox clinical trials. Radionics, incidentally, involves the use of an electrically operated receiver instead of the traditional human hand. As with all forms of alternative medicine there have been many 'quacks' operating in this field who have made it difficult for the honest practitioners.

spiritual healing
There are many branches of spiritual healing – divine healing, faith healing, psychic surgery and so on.
Suggested reading: *A Doctor Heals by Faith*, *The Reality of Spiritual Healing* by Christopher Woodward. Published by Hodder, 1959.

talisman therapy
Good luck charms designed to ward off evil and disease are still popular and many firms sell them in huge quantities. Whether the charm is a four-leaved clover or a copper bracelet, a herb pillow or a rabbit's foot, the 'placebo' effect is of prime importance – that is, if the purchaser believes in the charm there is a good chance that it will work.

Qualifications to look for

There are no official registers for the practitioners usually said to be working in the field of 'alternative' medicine. There are, however, many schools, colleges and other private establishments offering training courses and encouraging their graduates to add letters after their names. The following list of qualifications offered is by no means exhaustive.

BAc Graduate of the College of Traditional Chinese Acupuncture or the International College of Oriental Medicine

BEOA Member of the British and European Osteopathic Association

CO Graduate of Ecole Européenne d'Osteopathie

DAc Postgraduate of the International College of Oriental Medicine

DC Graduate of the Anglo-European College of Chiropractic, or the Oxfordshire School of Chiropractic

DO Graduate of British School of Osteopathy, College of Osteopathy and Manipulative Therapy and other establishments

LicAC Graduate of the British College of Acupuncture

MBAcA Member of the British Acupuncture Association

MCrOA Graduate of Cranial Osteopathic Association

MLCO Graduate of the London College of Osteopathy

MNIMH Graduate of the Tutorial School of Herbal Medicine at the National Institute of Medical Herbalists

MRadA Graduate of the School of Radionics in Ludlow, Shropshire

MSO Member of the Society of Osteopaths

MTAcS Member of the Traditional Acupuncture Society

ND DO Graduate of the British College of Naturopathy and Osteopathy

The Institutions

☐ *Health Service Hospitals, Homes and Clinics*

☐ *Private Hospitals, Homes and Clinics*

☐ Health Service Hospitals, Homes and Clinics

Hospitals

When the National Health Service was founded in 1948 one result was to bring together hospitals of many different kinds under a single administrative banner. There were short-stay private hospitals, long-stay charity hospitals, mental hospitals, eye hospitals, convalescent hospitals, geriatric hospitals, infectious disease hospitals, general hospitals, hospitals run by voluntary groups, hospitals run for the benefit of union or guild members and so on.

The original intention was to replace some of the older buildings with more modern edifices and to replace old-fashioned equipment with the latest and best in medical technology. Unhappily those good intentions did not pay the bills and the hospitals which exist in today's health service are often little or no better in structural terms than the hospitals which existed independently before 1948. Often the equipment within those hospitals is equally out of date.

The improvements which have been made have led to more rather than less patchiness within the hospital service in Britain; the area authorities which managed to put in their suggestions for new building programmes at times when government money was available now have well-equipped, well-built hospitals, while the authorities that timed their applications less fortunately still have to make do with crumbling buildings and out-dated equipment.

The patchiness is not simply geographical, however. There are great differences between the quality of buildings and equipment used for the care of acute, emergency medical cases and the quality of buildings and equipment used for the care of the chronic sick. Geriatric patients and psychiatric patients, for example, are often nursed in conditions which would be instantly recognizable by patients living in those same institutions half a century ago. The medical revolution has bypassed many of our chronic hospitals.

Which hospital?

The type of hospital to which a patient is admitted will depend on a number of very different factors. To begin with there must be a bed available and the hospital must be close enough to ensure that during the journey to the hospital there is a minimum amount of time for deterioration. The travelling factor is obviously most important for emergency cases, and patients whose problems are not medically urgent, and who are suffering from a disorder unusual enough to merit the attention of a super-specialist, may be advised to visit specialist units in hospitals many miles away from their own home district. (I use the term 'super-specialist' to define a consultant who offers a technical service to patients with a very narrow range of symptoms rather than to imply that the consultant is any way clinically superior to his colleagues.)

The type of disorder from which the patient suffers is naturally of importance. If there is a specialist hospital in the patient's own area which offers help to patients with a particular clinical problem, and the patient's GP considers that the hospital is suitable, then an approach will obviously be made to that institution. There are specialist geriatric, psychiatric and maternity hospitals in most parts of the country, for example.

If the problem is an acute one which needs immediate attention and there is no specialist hospital available locally then the GP will attempt to find a bed in the nearest general hospital. That hospital may be a teaching hospital (attached to a medical school) or any ordinary general hospital with facilities for admitting patients as emergencies.

The patient who needs emergency care and who has not been seen by a GP will usually be admitted to the nearest general hospital with a casualty department. During recent years changes in the health service have meant that not all local general hospitals accepting emergency admissions from GPs have casualty departments. The local ambulance service will know which hospitals have a casualty department and in an emergency, even if an ambulance is not required, the quickest way to find the address of the nearest casualty department is to telephone 999. Most ambulance station officers can give good directions to anyone travelling from a point within their own catchment area.

Note: Section 155 of the Road Traffic Act of 1972 entitles NHS hospitals to charge a fee for providing emergency treatment to people suffering from injuries caused by or arising out of road traffic accidents. Under the Act patients are liable to pay this fee if requested to do so. Official receipts can usually be obtained and insurance companies may pay the patient back.

Availability of hospital beds

Inside a general hospital patients are sorted out according to age, sex and medical status. Children under the age of 12 years are usually put onto special children's wards, while patients whose problems are considered mainly surgical will naturally be admitted to surgical wards. Other patients will be distributed around the hospital according to the availability of other specialist units. Any patient considered to be in need of very intensive care may be put into a special intensive care unit or intensive therapy unit where there will usually be a high concentration of sophisticated equipment and a high nurse-to-patient ratio. If there is a coronary care unit in the hospital any patient who has suffered a heart attack will be put in that unit for the first 24 or 48 hours of his hospital stay.

Patients who have been referred to hospital for non-urgent treatment will usually spend some time on a waiting list before being admitted. Admissions from the waiting list are known as 'cold' admissions. NHS lists reached an all-time high of 740,000 in March 1979; at the moment in Britain there are said to be about 650,000 patients awaiting hospital admission. (Some observers claim that this peak size for waiting lists occurred as a result of a hospital consultant's 'go slow' and that the apparent reduction in waiting list size since 1979 has not in fact resulted from any improvement in efficiency.) Most of the patients who are on waiting lists will have been seen by consultants in out-patient clinics but a small number will have been seen on domiciliary visits or as private patients. It used to be said that an easy way to jump the waiting list queue was to see a specialist privately and then be admitted to an NHS bed. Today, in theory, all patients being admitted to NHS hospital beds, whether they are being admitted to private wings (see p. 155) or NHS wards and whether they were seen in out-patient clinics or private consulting rooms, are supposed to go onto the same waiting list.

In practice there are several waiting lists rather than one single list; differentiation is theoretically based on clinical need. Recognizing that many people will have to wait months or even years for treatment, consultants try to arrange for individuals with urgent problems to be seen as soon as possible. Even dividing waiting lists in this way does not always prove effective, however, and in many hospitals there are now 'very urgent' waiting lists as well as 'urgent' and 'routine' lists. The place an individual patient has on a waiting list will usually depend on the consultant concerned but it may be a secretary's responsibility to maintain the list.

In most hospitals genuine attempts are made to keep all beds filled as often as possible (this increases the turnover of patients and helps to reduce the waiting list) but some beds do, of course, have to be kept open in hospitals which accept emergency admissions either from GPs alone or from GPs and their own casualty departments. (Incidentally, casualty departments are usually known to the administrators as accident and emergency units. Doctors and nurses refer to them as cas units.)

The problem facing those trying to keep the lists as short as possible and yet keep some beds available for emergency patients are such that the patient who agrees to be admitted at short notice may well find his waiting time reduced considerably.

Patients who insist on having two weeks' notice and who expect their own holiday dates to be honoured will, I'm afraid, have to wait a long time for NHS treatment.

On rare occasions patients admitted to hospital through the ordinary waiting list will find that there is no bed available. This may occur as a result of an appalling clerical error but it is far more likely to occur as a result of the bed being one of those filled by an unexpected influx of emergency patients. Some hospitals ask patients to telephone a few minutes before setting out for the hospital, just to confirm that there is an available bed, while other hospitals have administrative arrangements designed to ensure that this never happens twice to one patient.

In May 1981 a woman waiting for a hip operation was apparently told that she would have to wait 40 years. An MP who investigated found that lists varied enormously around the country. The suggestion was made that a computer bed bank be introduced to match patients waiting for operations with vacancies on waiting lists around the country. It has also been suggested that more mixed sex wards would help to reduce waiting lists. These are, however, still ideas for the future.

Day case units

Although most patients are admitted to a ward for a stay of at least a few days there is an increasing number of NHS hospitals which run 'day case units'. To cut costs and to increase further the turnover of patients, doctors arrange for patients with minor problems (such as small cysts needing removal, uncomplicated hernias needing repair and so on) to go into hospital in the early morning, to have whatever treatment is required, and to go home again within a few hours. At home the patient will usually be looked after by the district nurse who in turn will have the patient's GP to call on should any problems arise.

Although it is in the treatment of surgical patients that the use of day case units offers most hope to those hundreds of thousands of people on the national waiting lists (for even those patients with conditions which cannot be dealt with in a day case unit will benefit if the pressure on beds can be reduced), day case units do not only involve surgical patients. There have, in recent years, also been a number of experiments with special day hospitals for geriatric patients.

The theory behind the development of these special units is simple enough: the size of the elderly population in Britain is growing at a tremendous rate and many of these elderly folk are weak, frail and slightly disabled – they need some help if they are to survive. There is not enough public or private money around to provide geriatric hospitals, public nursing homes or sheltered accommodation for all the elderly people in need. Geriatric day hospitals, however, offer a degree of support at modest cost. For a sum which is relatively small old people can be transported from their own homes to these special units where they can eat, socialize and receive whatever basic nursing care may be required. Most geriatric day hospitals are supervised by hospital consultants but GPs are usually invited to recommend suitable patients.

GP hospitals

There is one other type of hospital service offered by the National Health Service which I have not mentioned yet and that is the general practitioner hospital.

A few years ago the trend among hospital architects and high level administrators was to advocate 'big is better' as a building policy. A number of enormous hospital complexes were planned, and some of them were built, but unfortunately the planners discovered that in practice things do not run quite as smoothly as they do in theory. It was found that the running costs for larger hospitals can be horrific and that nurses are often difficult to find since large hospitals have a reputation for being impersonal. As a result, some of the cottage hospitals which had been threatened with closure by previous administrations have been kept alive as GP hospitals.

There are obviously severe limitations on what can be done in a GP hospital but although major surgery is clearly a non-starter

147

there are other possibilities. For example, GP hospitals can be used as diagnostic centres and they are eminently suitable for minor surgery, for general nursing and convalescent care.

VD clinics

There is one branch of the hospital service which routinely sees patients who have not been referred by a general practitioner – that is the branch offering advice and information about sexually transmitted disorders. The specialists (known as venereologists) will almost always see any patient who turns up. The units where venereologists work may be called VD clinics or special clinics. Addresses and times of special clinics can be obtained from telephone directories, general practitioners, hospital switchboards and some public lavatories.

Involuntary admissions

Even though they may need hospital care some patients are unwilling to accept help.

Where the patient concerned is alert, mentally capable of making his or her own decisions, and not living in obviously unsuitable surroundings, there is nothing that anyone can do to force that patient to go into hospital. Members of some religious groups may strenuously resist attempts to admit them to hospital because of strong convictions that they hold. That is their right.

However, where there is good evidence that the individual concerned may be a danger either to himself or to others there are laws which can be invoked.

The Mental Health Act of 1959 is the most widely used piece of legislation. Where mentally ill patients have refused to go into hospital relatives or social workers may apply for their admission to be recommended by two medical practitioners. An application for admission to hospital for observation should be made under Section 25 of the Act. An application under Section 25 is good for a maximum of 28 days. Where longer term treatment in hospital is required and the patient is not willing to stay in hospital an application under Section 26 must be signed by two doctors.

In an emergency, one doctor can sign an application under Section 29 of the Mental Health Act but such an application is good for no more than 72 hours. Before that period has expired an application must be signed to convert the Section 29 to a Section 25 application.

These applications all concern patients who are thought to be mentally ill.

If a patient is thought to be living in entirely unsuitable surroundings and to be incapable of looking after himself properly for physical or mental reasons, a social worker and a medical practitioner can obtain a warrant from a Justice of the Peace to enter the individual's home and move him or her to a local hospital or other suitable institution for a period not exceeding 72 hours.

Tips for getting admitted to an NHS hospital quickly if your problem is non-urgent

1 See the consultant privately. Waiting lists for ordinary preliminary out-patient appointments often stretch to several weeks or even months. A private appointment (which will usually cost up to £25) should cut a considerable amount of time off this. You may also be put on a more urgent treatment list if you have seen the consultant privately.

2 Do not give a long list of dates when admission would not be convenient for you.

3 Give a telephone number and agree to go into hospital at short notice. Beds sometimes become available at a few hours' notice and patients known to be willing to drop

everything and rush to the hospital may be seen much sooner.

4 Telephone the consultant's secretary every week if you have been waiting for some time for your admission. There is not much point in telephoning your GP, unless there has been a substantial change in your clinical condition, since he has no control over hospital waiting lists. Plead with the consultant's secretary and she may be able to speed your admission. If you persist she may arrange for your admission to get you off her back.

Things they do to you in hospital and why

They wake you up at 6.00 a.m.

There is no clinical excuse for this barbaric custom. There are, however, two administrative excuses. First, the night nurses are expected to perform certain chores before the day nurses come on duty around 8.00 a.m. Those chores cannot be performed if the patients are asleep. And, second, most ward sisters like to get the routine chores out of the way before doctors start wandering around the hospital.

They shave you in intimate places and it itches for weeks afterwards

Patients who are destined for the operating table have to be prepared. Part of the preparation involves shaving the hair from the part of the body that is going to be the subject of attention. If the vagina or penis are likely to be involved the pubic hair may have to be removed. This is done simply to make it easier to clean the skin and to see what is what. A junior nurse or porter usually does the shaving.

They give you sleeping pills at night

Most people have a little difficulty in getting off to sleep at night in hospital. That is not unusual since few of us spend our nights sleeping in dormitories these days. Snoring patients, hospital plumbing, whispering nurses and the clank of bedpans can keep patients awake. It is important to stop taking sleeping pills when you go home if you can manage without but it is worth re-membering that it may take a day or two to get used to sleeping without a pharmaceutical aid.

But they wake you up to give you sleeping pills!

Sounds crazy and probably is but the argument nurses some-times offer is that the patient who does not need a pill earlier in the evening may wake up and need one later and then, having taken the pill in the middle of the night, will be difficult to rouse in the morning.

They seem obsessed with bowels

After surgery (particularly surgery on the intestines) medical and nursing staff like to know that the digestive tract is working normally. That is why they keep asking if you've 'passed wind' or 'had your bowels opened' and that is why they look so pleased when you have.

They make you stay in bed and complain if you crease the sheets

Some consultants get very crotchety if their patients are not in bed when they do their rounds. It is much easier to be dominant when your patient is dressed in pyjamas and horizontal than it is when your patient is sitting in his dressing-gown. Some ward sisters take it as a personal insult if the bedlinen does not look crisp and smart. There is no real logical explanation for these behavioural patterns but you are unlikely to be able to change the habits of a lifetime. Humour them as best you can.

They put a needle in your arm and leave it there connected up to a bottle

Drip-feeding patients is necessary for a number of reasons. The patient who cannot swallow or who cannot drink fluids the

What to take with you when you go into hospital

1 Any letter of introduction or explanation written by your own doctor

2 Nightdress or pyjamas

3 Dressing-gown and slippers

4 Box of paper tissues

5 Toilet bag with all the usual contents for an overnight stay

6 Make-up and cosmetic bag. (This item is optional for men)

7 A small silent bedside clock

8 A bag containing all the medicines you normally take. Or a list of them

9 Enough money to buy a newspaper, magazine and sweets

10 Books, magazines and notepaper and pencil

Do not take clothes (unless you have been specifically asked to do so), expensive jewellery of any kind (and that includes watches), or more than a couple of pounds in money

normal way will need feeding intravenously and the patient whose own intravenous fluids have become unbalanced for some reason will need a booster from a bottle. In addition to blood there is a wide variety of clear fluids available for drip-feeding patients. Putting drip needles into veins is a job usually left to house officers who tend to get very cross with patients who persist in dislodging them.

They starve you

If you are going to the operating theatre you will not be allowed to eat. You are starved simply to ensure that your stomach is as empty as possible while you are unconscious on the operating table. The patient with a full stomach may vomit and vomiting unconscious patients are a danger to themselves.

They make you get out of bed the day after the operation

Many of the more dangerous post-operative complications can be avoided by getting patients out of bed as soon as possible after they have returned to the ward. If they want you to get out of bed then do so!

They put a label on your wrist as though you were a piece of meat

Guard that label with your life. If it goes no one will know who you are and they may do things to you that you'll afterwards wish they hadn't done.

Other institutions run by the state

There are a number of long-term residential homes outside the hospital service but under the general auspices of the DHSS. Since most of the people living in them need physical support rather than specialized medical or nursing care such institutions as those offering accommodation to children in need, to the mentally subnormal, to the chronically disabled or to the elderly are run by local authorities through their social services departments and are usually staffed by social workers who have neither medical nor nursing training.

It is indeed important to understand that doctors have no authority at all over any of these homes and that admission lists are administered entirely by social workers. Applications for admission should usually be addressed to the local Director of Social Services.

The homes under most pressure are undoubtedly those offering accommodation to the elderly and, although local authority residential homes at present provide beds for some two-thirds of the 150,000 elderly people living in residential homes in Britain, there is little doubt that the available accommodation is greatly over-subscribed.

Social workers vetting applicants for admission to local authority old people's homes usually expect successful candidates to be able to support themselves physically, to be continent of both urine and faeces, to be mobile and coherent and to be generally suitable for accommodation which is, in theory at least, more akin to that in an old-fashioned seaside hotel than to that in a hospital of any kind. Residents have to pay towards the cost of their accommodation.

⊐ *Private Hospitals, Homes and Clinics*

Providing private medical care in Britain is a growing industry and the politically motivated attempts to end private medical care have failed quite miserably. Indeed it is now well known that many trade unionists who support publicly the political opposition to the provision of an alternative form of health care are personally subscribing to private health care organizations. A general discussion of private medical care within Britain and an account of the various insurance organizations offering cover can be found on pp. 26 and 318 respectively.

Private hospitals

Some NHS hospitals still have pay-beds where private patients can be looked after, and many have what are called 'amenity' beds. These are beds which are usually either in private single rooms or in small wards containing two or three beds and, while they may be used for the treatment of the very seriously ill, the mentally disordered, or the embarrassed socialist politician who does not want to go onto a public ward but who does not want to be seen in a private hospital, they are also sometimes made available to ordinary patients at a comparatively modest charge.

Private beds in NHS hospitals are only available to patients who are paying a specialist for private treatment but amenity beds may be made available to patients who are receiving NHS treatment. Inquiries about the availability of amenity beds should be addressed to the administrator of the local hospital; arrangements concerning private beds will usually be made by the patient's own consultant.

In addition to those health service hospitals which still offer private accommodation to patients there is now a growing number of hospitals which offer only private medical care. The *Directory of Private Hospitals and Health Services*, which is published by MMI Medical Market Information Ltd, contains a comprehensive list of the private hospitals in Britain. I have not included details of any specific private hospitals here for the simple but important reason that such hospitals do not admit patients who have not been referred by GPs. Other organizations which might offer information about private hospitals include the Association of Independent Hospitals, the Independent Hospital Group Ltd, and the Nuffield Nursing Homes Trust.

Advantages of private hospital treatment

1 Waiting lists are usually much shorter. This does not affect patients with genuinely urgent problems, but patients who might otherwise be put on 'cold' waiting lists will almost certainly benefit.

2 When going into hospital you can choose a time that is convenient to you rather than a time that is simply convenient to the hospital.

3 As an in-patient you will have a number of special perks: you may have a private bathroom; there will be more general privacy; there will be access to a telephone; visitors will be allowed freely, and so on.

4 The National Health Service benefits because some of the people who have already paid for NHS facilities (through their taxes) are effectively opting out and paying for treatment a second time. This must help to reduce general waiting times.

5 Any treatment you need will almost certainly be provided by the consultant who is looking after you.

Disadvantages of private hospital treatment

1 Private patients sometimes find that being in a private room for days on end can be lonely, even claustrophobic. Under some circumstances it can even be dangerous since unlike patients in a general ward, who are never out of sight of the nurses, patients in private rooms may collapse unseen.

2 If your problem is exceptional you will be better off in an NHS hospital where consultants have access to a wider range of skills and diagnostic services.

3 In a real emergency, health service general wards are usually better. It is sometimes physically difficult to get resuscitation equipment into a small private room.

4 The consultant who is looking after you is unlikely to be immediately available at all times. This means that there will not be any immediate access to medical care since consultants in private practice do not usually have juniors to cope with the day-to-day responsibilities.

Health farms and hydros

There is a growing number of health farms in Britain offering a wide range of services. A few offer medical care and have resident medical officers and nurses; the majority, however, concentrate on providing facilities designed to satisfy those needing extra exercise and dietary assistance.

The hydros are so called because they offer their clients hydro-therapy – a rather smart term for any form of treatment which involves water and which may include bathing in it or simply drinking it.

Both health farms and hydros usually offer their clients a selection of beauty treatments to choose from.

The cost of staying in a health farm or at a hydro can be extremely high and the customer whose main desire is to have a quiet restful few days away from the hurly burly of city life might do better in all respects to find a quiet country hotel.

There is in addition one other very cheap way to get away from it all and that is to spend ten days at the Common Cold Unit in the Wiltshire countryside. The staff at the Cold Unit, who have been researching the ways in which people catch colds for some years now, will look after you entirely free of charge and will pay travelling expenses and pocket money as well. Over 400 people a year visit the Unit and many find it an excellent centre for relaxing, studying and hiding away from the world. The address for those interested is: The Clinical Administrator, Common Cold Unit, Havard Hospital, Coombe Road, Salisbury SP2 8BW.

Nursing homes and rest homes

The title 'nursing home' is used to describe institutions offering widely different qualities of care and service and it is important when contemplating making use of any such institution to decide exactly what sort of service is required.

At the top end of the range there are nursing homes which are effectively offering private hospital facilities. Some have their own operating theatres, full-time medical staff and a wide range of medical equipment. At the other end of the scale there are the converted private houses which offer accommodation for a small number of mobile old people. These homes are really no different from guest houses or small private hotels. The fees charged by nursing homes should obviously reflect the quality of care and service provided but there are some proprietors offering very basic facilities and charging exorbitant prices.

A number of independent organizations maintain lists of nursing homes and rest homes which should serve as a useful guide to anyone looking for such accommodation. The Registered Nursing Home Association and the Registered Rest Home Association both represent a number of such institutions, but the best complete directory that I know of is the *Directory of Private*

Hospitals and Health Services which lists the addresses of about 150 hospitals, and several thousand nursing, rest and private homes offering accommodation.

Although there is much overlapping between the type of service provided by nursing homes and rest homes there are some theoretical differences.

Officially a nursing home is defined as any place used for the reception and nursing of persons suffering from any illness and, according to the Nursing Homes Act of 1975, all nursing homes have to be registered with local authorities, with premises and staff having to satisfy specific regulations. There is, as you might expect, much legislation governing the availability of wash basins, curtains and fire escapes and a doctor or nurse has to be available, but although these regulations do go some way towards helping define the minimum quality of care in a nursing home there is not, nor can there be, any legislative control ensuring that nursing homes provide their residents with kindness or good nursing care.

Rest homes, sometimes known as private homes and sometimes also, confusingly, known as nursing homes, have to be registered with local authorities under the National Assistance Act of 1948 and they are officially intended to provide accommodation for the disabled and the elderly. Private homes do not have to have a qualified nurse in attendance.

A large number of the nursing homes and rest homes in existence are run by charitable organizations and intended to provide temporary or permanent accommodation for individuals suffering from specific disabilities. A list of some of the organizations which deal exclusively with individuals suffering from particular conditions can be found on pp. 174ff. Many of the organizations listed there either own or have access to specialist nursing homes and rest homes. General practitioners will have details of and access to local homes in particular areas of the country.

Many of these institutions are, however, not run by charitable organizations but on a purely private basis by individuals or companies hoping to make a profit. This is a perfectly laudable motive, of course, as long as the individuals operating the home maintain a sense of perspective. Acknowledging that the majority of these homes cater largely if not exclusively for the elderly I have prepared three checklists, describing some of the advantages and disadvantages of nursing and rest homes for the elderly, and providing potential clients with a guide designed to enable them to make a wise choice.

Advantages of nursing home care for the elderly

1   Basic needs will be met regularly. Cleaning and cooking and other domestic chores will be tended to by able-bodied aides. Maintenance and service problems disappear entirely.

2   Loneliness is banished. Many of the people living in nursing homes are widowed, unmarried or childless; if they had to live alone they would rarely see other people.

3   Pressures on small family units can be avoided. If an elderly relative is looked after in a small house the physical, mental, social and economic problems can be considerable. It is usually the woman in the household who suffers most as she struggles to satisfy the needs of all those in her care.

4   When a nursing home is chosen carefully the benefits to the individual in terms of intellectual stimulation can be considerable. A major problem for the elderly is coming to terms with the relative lack of purpose which so often accompanies old age. In a good home this problem can be minimized.

5   Freeing family members from purely physical responsibilities means that stronger emotional ties can develop more easily. It is easier for all concerned to enjoy one another's company when duties and responsibilities are kept to an acceptable level.

6   When professional nursing care is needed on a permanent basis it is usually easier and sometimes cheaper to obtain it in a purpose-built institution.

Disadvantages of nursing home care for the elderly

1 There are badly run nursing homes where residents have to fit the system and where there is considerable risk that all individual charms will be subordinated to the needs of the institution.

2 If abandoned in a nursing home many elderly people feel unwanted. Relatives may suffer from feelings of guilt.

3 The costs of nursing home care can be considerable, and, if the extent of the care that can be afforded is not determined at the outset, problems may arise when the money runs out.

4 In a badly run home old people may be ignored, mistreated and exploited. Staff may be overworked and undertrained, food may be inadequate in quantity and lacking in nutritional value and private property may be stolen or misused. In order to reduce the amount of work, staff in bad homes encourage residents to be apathetic rather than independent and may even provide regular sedatives in order to keep problem patients quiet. There is no single criterion which can be used to help potential residents and their relatives decide whether or not a nursing home offers good or bad service. Registration simply means that the home's owners have satisfied certain basic criteria. The atmosphere in a home is, however, much more important and it is for this reason that I suggest that all potential residents should visit a home before going to stay there.

Points to remember when choosing a private home for an old person

1 Decide whether a nursing home, rest home or hotel would be most suitable.

2 Check that the home you choose is properly registered.

3 Make sure that you understand exactly what is included in the weekly cost and what charges are made for any extras.

If a long-term stay is contemplated the availability of funds must be considered carefully.

4 Visit the home and ask to be allowed to look round. Certain cosmetic work can be done to improve the appearance of a home when visitors are due but it is not possible to do anything about ingrained dirt or the too common all-pervading smell of stale urine.

5 Find out what arrangements are made for medical care. In a nursing home there should be a qualified nurse on duty at all times. In any establishment for the care of the elderly there should obviously be arrangements for calling for medical help. Are residents allowed to have a doctor of their choice or do they have to register with a particular doctor?

6 Ask whether residents can take their own furniture into the home. And find out the rules about pets. Are newspapers delivered? Are private TV sets and radios allowed?

7 Find out what the rules about visitors are. There really shouldn't be any strict rules although it is quite reasonable to ask visitors to wait if meals are being served. Some nursing homes and rest homes keep accommodation free for visitors wishing to stay overnight.

8 See what sort of call system is available if the home is supposed to be suitable for the bed-ridden. A properly equipped nursing home should have call buttons by the side of each bed.

9 If there are prefabricated buildings in the garden check to see that there are extra bathrooms and toilet facilities to cope with the added number of residents.

10 If room sharing is a possibility find out who the other occupant of the room is likely to be.

11 Remember that all private nursing homes are run for profit. There is nothing wrong with that unless the owner is trying to make too much money too quickly.

Screening clinics

Most health care facilities are designed to cater for the sick. Screening clinics, on the other hand, are intended to be used by the healthy. The theory behind their evolution is simple enough.

There are certain medical tests sometimes done routinely as part of a thorough medical examination to provide clear evidence of the existence of a developing disease process.

A blood pressure check, for example, will show the existence of high blood pressure long before the patient himself is aware of the existence of any problem. An examination of the female breasts will show the presence of any lumps long before such abnormalities would be noticed as unusual. A urine examination will show the presence of excess sugar, and therefore hint strongly at the possibility of diabetes, some time before the patient has any clinical symptoms of diabetes. Those are three of the tests commonly done at a screening clinic, but there are others.

The rising demand for screening checks has not, unfortunately, been accompanied by any increase in the facilities within the health services designed to accommodate such a demand. Health service doctors, whether they are working within the hospital service or in the community, are contracted to provide general medical care for the sick. They are not under obligation to provide the healthy with any sort of care or advice. Indeed, the demands within the NHS are such that attempts to offer screening checks would only produce a further reduction in the quality of the service available to the sick.

The demand for screening clinics has, however, been met by the private sector and there are today a good many private organizations offering screening checks. BUPA, for example, estimate that in the last ten years they have screened 200,000 individuals and that their present screening programme involves 30,000 people a year. A number of other private organizations around the country offer similar programmes which may or may not include a physical examination. The cost of a health screening examination is likely to be approximately £100. It may be considerably more.

Whether or not screening clinics offer a clinically worthwhile service justifying such heavy expenditure is another matter. A government-financed survey concluded in 1979 that regular screening examinations are expensive and ineffective, and one eminent cardiologist has been reported as saying that there are only two things worth doing at a check-up: one is to take the blood pressure, and treat it if necessary, and the other is to find out how much the patient smokes and try and stop him smoking if appropriate.

Certainly it can be argued that having an annual screening check is about as useful as getting a bank statement once a year. You do not really learn much about yourself either way and you certainly are not protected from any potential disaster which may loom ahead. On the other hand although having a screening check may be expensive it cannot do any harm to have one.

If you want a check-up and you cannot afford £100 then see p. 306 for my home screening tests. In addition you might find that your own doctor will be prepared to check your blood pressure next time you make a routine visit to the surgery. Take a sample of urine with you and he will probably be happy to test that for you too. Women can get cervical smears done in local authority clinics or by general practitioners; they can learn to examine their own breasts once a month (see p. 46 in my book *Aspirin or Ambulance?* published by Jill Norman).

The Organizations

☐ *Statutory and Professional*

☐ *Private and Voluntary*

☐ *Statutory and Professional*

A to Z directory of statutory and professional organizations

Health care is big business which involves many hundreds of thousands of employees and many millions of pounds. Inevitably, therefore, a large number of organizations exist to administer the health service and to look after the interests of professionals in specific groups.

The list which follows includes details of the governing bodies of the professions usually regarded as 'supplementary to medicine'. Anyone interested in following a career in one of these supplementary professions, or indeed in medicine itself, should write for basic information to the appropriate organization.

Association of Anaesthetists of Great Britain and Ireland
Tavistock House South, Tavistock Square, London WC1H 9JP

Association of the British Pharmaceutical Industry
162 Regent Street, London W1R 6DD

Association of Chief Administrators of Health Authorities
The National Hospital for Nervous Diseases, Queen Square, London WC1N 3BG

Association of Clinical Biochemists
30 Russell Square, London WC1B 5DT

Association of Health Care Information and Medical Records Officers
16 Beacon Hill, Dormansland, Lingfield, Surrey RH7 6RH

Association of Health Sector and Unit Administrators
General Hospital, Hospital Road, Port Talbot, West Glamorgan SA12 6PD

Association of Independent Hospitals and Kindred Organizations
14 Fitzroy Square, London W1

Association of Medical Secretaries
Tavistock House South, Tavistock Square, London WC1H 9LN

Association of National Health Service Supplies Officers
Signal House, Lyon Road, Harrow, Middlesex HA1 2EL

Association of Nurse Administrators
13 Grosvenor Place, London SW1X 7EN

Association of Optical Practitioners
233 Blackfriars Road, London SE1 8NW
(represents ophthalmic opticians)

Association of Scientific, Technical and Managerial Staffs (ASTMS)
10–26a Jamestown Road, London NW1 7DT

Association of Sexual and Marital Therapists
79 Harley Street, London W1N 1DE

British Acupuncture Association and Register Ltd
34 Alderney Street, London SW1V 4EU

British Association of Manipulative Medicine Ltd
22 Harley Street, London W1N 1AA

British Association of Occupational Therapists
20 Rede Place, Bayswater, London W2 4TU

British Association of Social Workers
16 Kent Street, Birmingham B5 6RD

British Dental Association
63 Wimpole Street, London W1M 8AL
(looks after the interests of the dental profession)

British Dietetic Association Inc
305 Daimler House, Paradise Street, Birmingham B1 2BJ

British Homoeopathic Association
27a Devonshire Street, London W1N 1RJ

British Medical Association
BMA House, Tavistock Square, London WC1H 9JP
(one of the oldest, largest and most powerful medical trade unions; includes
many, but by no means all, British doctors among its members)

British Naturopathic and Osteopathic Association
Frazer House, 6 Netherhall Gardens, London NW3 5RR

British Optical Association
10 Knaresborough Place, London W1Y 2DT

British Osteopathic Association
8–10 Boston Place, London NW1 6QH

British Psychological Society
18–19 Albermarle Street, London W1X 4DN
(looks after the interests of psychology and psychologists)

British Society of Audiology
Harvest House, 62 London Road, Reading RG1 5AS

Central Midwives Board
39 Harrington Gardens, London SW7 4JY

Chartered Society of Physiotherapy
14 Bedford Row, London WC1R 4ED
(training, examining and registering body for physiotherapists)

Chiropractic Medical Association
51 Canford Cliffs Road, Poole, Dorset BH13 7AQ

College of Speech Therapists
6 Lechmere Road, London NW2 5BU
(administration and registration of speech therapy and speech therapists)

Committee on Safety of Medicines
Finsbury Square House, 33–37a Finsbury Square, London EC2B 2ZS

Confederation of Health Service Employees (COHSE)
Glen House, High Street, Banstead, Surrey SM7 2LH
(specialist trade union for NHS employees; includes medical and non-medical staff)

Council for Professions Supplementary to Medicine
184 Kennington Park Road, London SE11 4BT
(the eight types of professional officially recognized as 'supplementary' to medicine are: chiropodists, dieticians, medical laboratory technicians, occupational therapists, orthoptists, physiotherapists, radiographers and remedial gymnasts; the Council looks after the registration of members of these professions)

Department of Health and Social Security
Alexander Fleming House, Elephant and Castle, London SE1 6BY
(centre of the health service)

Fellowship for Freedom in Medicine
86 Harley Street, London W1N 1AE
(promotes private practice and supports private medical practitioners)

General Council and Register of Osteopaths
16 Buckingham Gate, London SW1E 6LB

General Dental Council
37 Wimpole Street, London W1M 8DQ
(maintains a list of qualified dentists and is in charge of discipline for the profession)

General Medical Council
44 Hallam Street, London W1N 6AE
(maintains a list of qualified and registered medical practitioners, supervises medical education, and is in official charge of the profession's ethical standards; its disciplinary hearings provide the popular newspapers with many inches of copy)

General Nursing Council for England and Wales
23 Portland Place, London W1A 1BA
(conducts examinations for nurses and maintains a register of qualified nurses)

General Nursing Council for Scotland
5 Darnaway Street, Edinburgh EH3 6DP
(looks after nurses and nursing in Scotland)

General Optical Council
41 Harley Street, London W1N 2DJ
(does for opticians what the General Medical Council does for doctors)

Health Education Council
78 New Oxford Street, London WC1A 1AH
(organizes campaigns and publishes leaflets designed to help promote good
health)

Health Visitors Association
36 Eccleston Square, London SW1V 1PF

Hospital Consultants and Specialists Association
The Old Court House, London Road, Ascot, Berks SL5 7EN
(represents interests of a large number of specialists – in competition with the
BMA)

Institute of Health Service Administrators
75 Portland Place, London W1N 4AN

Institute of Medical Laboratory Technology
12 Queen Anne Street, London W1M 0AU

Junior Hospital Doctors Association
199b Temple Chambers, Temple Avenue, London EC4Y 0JB
(looks after the interests of junior hospital doctors – in competition with the
BMA)

King's Fund Centre
126 Albert Street, London NW1 7NF
(arranges discussions and publications relating to the health service)

Medical Defence Union
3 Devonshire Place, London W1N 2EA
(the oldest and largest medical defence organization in the world; doctors and
dentists pay an annual premium and are provided with legal aid and financial
support if sued by unhappy patients)

Medical Practitioners Union
10–26 Jamestown Road, London NW1 7BY
(a medical trade union – in competition with the BMA)

Medical Protection Society
50 Hallam Street, London W1N 6DE (offers a similar service to the MDU)

Medical Research Council
20 Park Crescent, London W1N 4AL

National Association of Certificated Nursery Nurses
158 Victoria Rise, London SW4 0NW

National Association of Health Authorities in England and Wales
Park House, 40 Edgbaston Park Road, Birmingham B15 2RT

National Association of Voluntary Help Organizers
High Royds Hospital, Bradford Road, Menston, Ilkley, West Yorks LS29 6AQ

National Institute for Social Work
Mary Ward House, 5–7 Tavistock Place, London WC1H 9SS

National Pharmaceutical Union
Mallinson House, 321 Chase Road, London N14 6JN
(looks after the interests of proprietor pharmacists)

Pharmaceutical Society of Great Britain
1 Lambeth High Street, London SE1 7JN
(looks after the interests of pharmacists)

Physiotherapists Association
Heath House, 284 Broadway, Bexleyheath, Kent DA6 8AJ
(registered trade union)

Register of Approved Private Hospitals and Nursing Homes
3 Moor Lane, Budleigh Salterton, Devon EX9 6PW

Royal College of General Practitioners
14 Princes Gate, London SW7 1PU

Royal College of Midwives
15 Mansfield Street, London W1M 0BE

Royal College of Nursing
1a Henrietta Place, London W1M 0AB
(looks after the interests of nurses)

Royal College of Pathologists
2 Carlton House Terrace, London SW1Y 5AF

Royal College of Physicians of Edinburgh
9 Queen Street, Edinburgh EH2 1JQ

Royal College of Physicians of Ireland
6 Kildare Street, Dublin

Royal College of Physicians of London
11 St Andrew's Place, Regent's Park, London NW1 4LE

Royal College of Physicians and Surgeons of Glasgow
242 St Vincent Street, Glasgow G2 5RJ

Royal College of Psychiatrists
17 Belgrave Square, London SW1X 8PG

Royal College of Surgeons of Edinburgh
18 Nicolson Street, Edinburgh EH8 9DW

Royal College of Surgeons of England
35 Lincoln's Inn Fields, London WC2A 3PN

Royal College of Surgeons in Ireland
123 St Stephen's Green, Dublin 2

Royal Society of Medicine
1 Wimpole Street, London W1M 8AE
(has one of the best medical libraries in the world; members and fellows do not
pass any entrance examination)

Scottish Council for Health Education
Health Education Centre, 21 Lansdowne Crescent, Edinburgh EH12 5EJ

Socialist Medical Association
14–16 Bristol Street, Birmingham B5 7AA

Society of Administrators of Family Practitioner Services
42 West Cliff, Preston, Lancs PR1 8HQ

Society of Chiropodists
8 Wimpole Street, London W1M 8BX

Society of Family Practitioner Committees
Sutton New Road, Erdington, Birmingham B23 6TR

Society of Opticians
63 Great Cumberland Place, Bryanston Square, London W1H 7LJ

Society of Radiographers
14 Upper Wimpole Street, London W1M 8BN

Society of Remedial Gymnasts
c/o Northampton Town FC, County Ground, Abington Avenue,
Northampton NN1 4PS

Union of Speech Therapists
29 High Street, Great Bookham, Leatherhead, Surrey KT23 4AA

World Health Organization
20 Avenue Appia, 1211 Geneva, Switzerland
(the WHO's working budget for 1982–83 is an impressive $468,900,000)

□ Private and Voluntary

In addition to the large number of officially backed organizations offering advice and help to those in need of general support or specific information, there are very many unofficial and voluntary organizations. Some of these groups are well financed and employ dozens of professionally trained workers; others really do work on a very small budget and rely entirely on volunteers both for practical work and for administrative help. Some of these organizations are designed to offer advice and help to anyone in need while others are founded and run simply to help provide information for patients suffering from specific, well-defined disorders. Many of these small, specific organizations are themselves run by patients or their relatives and the quality of advice available is usually very high indeed.

These organizations offer patients and their relatives more than simple, practical help (valuable though that may be); they also offer encouragement and moral support. I heartily recommend that anyone who suffers from a specific chronic ailment or who is closely related to someone who does should join the appropriate organization.

The list which follows here is by no means comprehensive. There are many thousands of voluntary organizations in Britain and each year some weak ones disappear and some new ones appear. I have tried to prepare a comprehensive list which will enable any individual to find a starting point so, for example, anyone contacting one of the major organizations for the blind or the deaf will be able to obtain from that source details of other organizations offering support to the blind or deaf. Listing all the residential homes and other charities would take up a disproportionate amount of space in this book.

There are several points which are worth making about these voluntary organizations.

1 When writing to a voluntary organization for information do send a stamped addressed envelope.

2 Do remember that addresses of voluntary organizations change quite frequently as one honorary secretary hands over to another. Your letter may have to be forwarded and so delays are not unknown. If you do not receive a reply from one organization there may well be another group listed here which offers a similar range of services.

3 Please remember that all voluntary organizations need support from people like you in order to give advice to people like you. Most, if not all, of the organizations included in the following list will enthusiastically welcome offers of money or practical help. There are visits to be made, newsletters to be prepared and printed, meetings to be arranged and funds to be raised.

I would be very interested to know of new voluntary organizations that are being set up. Please write to me about them c/o Thames and Hudson, 30 Bloomsbury Street, London WC1B 3QP.

A to Z directory of private and voluntary organizations

The Action Against Allergy Association
43 The Downs, London SW20 8HG

Action on Smoking and Health (ASH)
27–35 Mortimer Street, London W1N 7RJ

Adoption Resource Exchange
11 Southwark Street, London SE1 1RQ

Age Concern
Bernard Sunley House, 60 Pitcairn Road, Mitcham, Surrey CR4 3LL

Al-Anon Family Groups
61 Great Dover Street, London SE1 4YF
(support and friendship for friends and relatives of alcoholics)

Albany Trust
16–20 Strutton Ground, London SW1P 2HP
(helps sexual minorities)

Albino Fellowship
15 Goukscroft Park, Ayr KA7 4DS
(provides encouragement, support and information for patients and their families)

Alcoholics Anonymous
Box 154, 11 Redcliffe Gardens, London SW10 9BQ

Anorexic Aid
Gravel House, Copthall Corner, Chalfont St Peter, Gerrards Cross, Bucks SL9 0BZ

Arthritis and Rheumatism Council for Research
Faraday House, 8–10 Charing Cross Road, London WC2H 0HN

Association for All Speech Impaired Children
347 Central Markets, Smithfield, London EC1A 9LH

Association of British Adoption and Fostering Agencies
4 Southampton Row, London WC1B 4AA

Association for Children with Heart Disorders
11 Millthorne Avenue, Clitheroe, Lancs BB7 2LE

Association for Children with Learning Disabilities
27 Hampton Road, Folly Hill, Farnham, Surrey GU9 0DQ

Association to Combat Huntington's Chorea
Lyndhurst, Lower Hampton Road, Sunbury on Thames, Middlesex TW16 5PR

Association of Disabled Professionals
The Stables, 73 Pound Road, Banstead, Surrey SM7 2HU

Association of Parents of Vaccine Damaged Children
2 Church Street, Shipston-on-Stour, Warwicks CV36 4AP

Association for Postnatal Illness
7 Gowan Avenue, London SW6 6RH

Association for Research into Restricted Growth
2 Mount Court, 81 Central Hill, London SE19 1BS

Association for Spina Bifida and Hydrocephalus
Tavistock House North, Tavistock Square, London WC1H 9HJ

Association for Stammerers
86 Blackfriars Road, London SE1 8HA

Asthma Research Council
12 Pembridge Square, London W2 4EH

Asthma Society *see* Asthma Research Council

Back Pain Association
Grundy House, Somerset Road, Teddington, Middlesex TW11 8TD

Dr Barnardos
Tanners Lane, Barkingside, Ilford, Essex IG6 1QG
(provides care and treatment of children in need)

Battered Wives *see* Womens Aid Federation

Beaumont Society
Box BM 5084, London WC1N 3XX
(organization to offer advice and information to transsexuals)

The Birth Centre
188 Old Street, London EC1V 9BP

British Association for the Retarded
117 Golden Lane, London EC1Y 0TJ

British Association of Retired Persons
1 Albyn Place, Edinburgh EH2 4NG

British Association for Service to the Elderly (which includes the
Geriatric Care Association)
60 Pitcairn Road, Mitcham, Surrey CR4 3LL

British Diabetic Association
10 Queen Anne Street, London W1M 0BD

British Dyslexia Association
4 Hobart Place, London SW1W 0HU

British Epilepsy Association
Crowthorne House, New Wokingham Road, Wokingham, Berks RG11 3AY

British Kidney Patient Association
Oakhanger Place, Bordon, Hants

British Leprosy Relief Association (LEPRA)
Fairfax House, Causton Road, Colchester, Essex CO1 1PU

British Limbless Ex-Servicemen's Association
Frankland Moor House, 185–187 High Road, Romford, Essex RM6 6NA

British Migraine Association
Evergreen, Ottermead Lane, Ottershaw, Chertsey, Surrey KT16 0HJ

British Polio Fellowship
Bell Close, West End Road, Ruislip, Middlesex HA4 6LP

British Pregnancy Advisory Service
PO Box 54, Austy Manor, Stratford Road, Wootton Wawen, Solihull,
West Midlands B95 6BX
(and see local telephone directory)

British Red Cross Society
9 Grovesnor Crescent, London SW1X 7EJ
(offers wide range of services to those in need)

British Retinitis Pigmentosa Society
24 Palmer Close, Redhill, Surrey RH1 4BX

British Rheumatism and Arthritis Association
6 Grovesnor Crescent, London SW1X 7EP

British Society for Music Therapy
48 Lanchester Road, London N6 4TA

British Tay-Sachs Foundation
c/o Hospital for Sick Children, Great Ormond Street, London WC1N 3JH

British Thoracic & Tuberculosis Association (TB)
30 Britten Street, London SW3 6NN

British Tinnitus Association
c/o RNID, 105 Gower Street, London WC1E 6AH

Brittle Bone Society
63 Byron Crescent, Dundee DD3 6SS

Brook Advisory Centres
233 Tottenham Court Road, London W1P 9AE
(has centres around the country; for pregnancy tests, contraception,
abortion, etc)

Campaign for Homosexual Equality
42a Formosa Street, London W9 2JP

Campaign for the Mentally Handicapped
96 Portland Place, London W1N 3HD

Cancer After Care and Rehabilitation Society *see* CARE

Cancer Information Association
2nd Floor, Marigold House, Carfax, Oxford OX1 1EF

Cardiac Spare Parts Club
10 Duke Street, Little Common, Bexhill-on-Sea, East Sussex TN39 4JG
(for patients who have undergone major heart surgery)

CARE
Lodge Cottage, Church Lane, Timsbury, Bath, Avon BA3 1LF
(the Cancer After Care and Rehabilitation Society; offers advice and help to
cancer sufferers and their families)

Centre for Spastic Children
61 Cheyne Walk, London SW3 5LX

Chest, Heart & Stroke Association
Tavistock House North, Tavistock Square, London WC1H 9JE

Child Poverty Action Group
1 Macklin Street, London WC2B 5NH

Children's Heart Circle in Wales
48 Insole Grove East, Cardiff CF5 2HP
(support for Welsh children suffering from heart disease)

Citizens Rights Office
1 Macklin Street, London WC2B 5NH
(offers advice on all sorts of private and public liabilities)

Claimants Unions
44 Havelock Road, Handsworth, Birmingham B20 3LR
(runs advice groups for people on social security)

Coeliac Society of the United Kingdom
PO Box 181, London NW2 2QY

Colostomy Welfare Group
2nd Floor, 38–39 Eccleston Square, London SW1V 1PB

Committee of Sexual Problems of the Disabled
183 Queensway, London W2 5HL

Community Service Volunteers
237 Pentonville Road, London N1 9NJ
(short-term full-time volunteers are found work)

Council and Care for the Elderly (Elderly Invalid's Fund)
10 Fleet Street, London EC4Y 1AU

Crossroads Care Attendant Scheme Trust
11 Whitehall Road, Rugby, Warwicks CV21 3AQ
(a charitable trust specializing in the provision of people with nursing experience
who can help care for the disabled of all kinds at home)

177

CRUSE
The Charter House, Richmond, Surrey TW9 2DF
(organization for widows and widowers)

Cystic Fibrosis Research Trust
5 Blyth Road, Bromley, Kent BR1 3RS

Depressives Associated
19 Merley Ways, Wimborne Minster, Dorset BH21 1QN

Disabled Drivers Association
The Hall, Ashwellthorpe, Norwich NR16 1EX

Disabled Drivers Motor Club
9 Park Parade, Gunnersbury Avenue, London W3 9BD

Disabled Living Foundation
346 Kensington High Street, London W14 8NS
(keeps up-to-date lists of manufacturers and stockists of equipment for the
disabled)

Down's Children's Association
Mr L. Cordukes, Quinton Community Centre, Ridgacre Road, Quinton,
Birmingham B32 2TW

The Dyslexia Institute
133 Gresham Road, Staines, Middlesex TW18 2AJ
(specializes in the teaching and training of dyslexic children)

Equipment for the Disabled
2 Foredown Drive, Portslade, Brighton BN4 2BB

Family Planning Association
27 Mortimer Street, London W1
(and see local telephone directory)

Food Allergy Association
27 Ferringham Lane, Ferring by Sea, Worthing, West Sussex BN12 5NB

Foundation for the Study of Infant Deaths
4–5 Grosvenor Place, London SW1X 7HD

Friedrich's Ataxia Group
12c Worplesdon Road, Guildford, Surrey GU2 6RW

Gamblers Anonymous
17 Blantyre Street, London SW10 0DT

Gardens for the Disabled Trust
Headcorn Manor, Headcorn, Kent TN27 9NP

Gay Switchboard
(offers advice to homosexuals (01)837-7324; lesbians (01)837-8602)

Gingerbread
35 Wellington Street, London WC2E 7BN
(for single-parent families)

Haemophilia Society
PO Box 9, 16 Trinity Street, London SE1 1DE

Helen Arkell Dyslexia Centre
14 Crondace Road, London SW6 4BB

Help the Aged
32 Dover Street, London W1A 2AP

Hyperactive Children's Grove
59 Meadowside, Angmering, Near Littlehampton, West Sussex BN16 4BW

The Ileostomy Association of Great Britain and Ireland
Ambleside House, Chobham, Woking, Surrey GU24 8PZ

International Glaucoma Association
King's College Hospital, Denmark Hill, London SE5 9RS

Invalid Children's Aid Association
126 Buckingham Palace Road, London SW1W 9SB

La Leche League
Box BM 3424, London WC1V 6XX
(information and advice for mothers; help with breastfeeding problems)

Leukaemia Society
45 Craigmoor Avenue, Bournemouth, Dorset BH8 9LW

LIFE
35 Kenilworth Road, Leamington Spa, Warwicks CV32 6JG
(anti-abortion group; offers support and advice)

Lifeline
39 Victoria Street, London SW1H 0EE
(advice for unintentionally pregnant women who do not want an abortion)

Marie Curie Memorial Foundation
124 Sloane Street, London SW1X 9BP
(runs homes for and offers advice to cancer patients of all kinds)

Marie Stopes House
108 Whitfield Street, London W1P 5RU
(contraception and abortion etc.)

Mastectomy Advisory Service
40 Eglantine Avenue, Belfast BT9 6DX

Mastectomy Association
1 Colworth Road, Croydon, Surrey CR0 7AD

Medic Alert Foundation
9 Hanover Street, London W1R 9HF

Meet-a-Mum Association
26a Cumnor Hill, Oxford OX2 9HA
(helps women suffering from post-natal depression etc.)

179

Mental After Care Association
110 Jermyn Street, London SW1Y 6HB

Mental Health Foundation
8 Wimpole Street, London W1M 8HY

Migraine Trust
45 Great Ormond Street, London WC1N 3HD

MIND (National Association for Mental Health)
22 Harley Street, London W1N 2ED

Mothers Union
24 Tufton Street, London SW1P 3RB

Multiple Sclerosis Action Group (ARMS)
71 Grays Inn Road, London WC1X 8TR

Multiple Sclerosis Society of Great Britain and Northern Ireland
286 Munster Road, London SW6 6AP

Muscular Dystrophy Group of Great Britain and Myasthenia Gravis
Nattrass House, 35 Macaulay Road, London SW4 0QP

National Ankylosing Spondylitis Society
The Royal National Hospital for Rheumatic Diseases, Upper Borough Walls,
Bath, Avon BA1 1RL

National Association for the Childless
318 Summer Lane, Birmingham B19 3RL

National Association for Deaf/Blind and Rubella Handicapped
164 Cromwell Lane, Coventry CV4 8AP

National Association for Gifted Children
1 South Audley Street, London W1Y 5DQ

National Association of Laryngectomy Clubs
30 Dorset Square, London NW1 6QJ

National Association for the Relief of Paget's Disease
Ann Stansfield, 413 Middleton Road, Rhodes, Middleton,
Manchester M24 4QZ

National Association for the Welfare of Children in Hospital
7 Exton Street, London SE1 8UE
(advice and help for young patients and their parents)

National Bureau for Handicapped Students
Thomas Coram Foundation, 40 Brunswick Square, London WC1N 1AZ

National Childbirth Trust
9 Queensborough Terrace, London W2 3TB
(provides ante-natal classes for expectant mothers)

National Corporation for the Care of Old People
Nuffield Lodge, Regent's Park, London NW1 4RS

National Council on Alcoholism
3 Grosvenor Crescent, London SW1X 7EE

National Council for One Parent Families
255 Kentish Town Road, London NW5 21X

National Council for the Single Woman and her Dependants Ltd
29 Chilworth Mews, London W2 3RG

National Council of Social Service
26 Bedford Square, London WC1B 3HU

National Deaf Children's Society
31 Gloucester Place, London W1H 4EA

National Eczema Society
5–7 Tavistock Place, London WC1H 9SN

National Federation of Women's Institutes
39 Eccleston Street, London SW1W 9NT

National Housewives Register
Gants Mill, Bruton, Somerset BA10 0DB
(encourages stimulating discussions and meetings for lonely or bored women)

National Marriage Guidance Council
Herbert Gray College, Little Church Street, Rugby, Warwicks CV21 3AP

National Schizophrenia Fellowship
78–79 Victoria Road, Surbiton, Surrey KT6 4JT

National Society for Autistic Children
1a Golders Green Road, London NW11 8EA

National Society for Cancer Relief
30 Dorset Square, London NW1 6QL

National Society for Epilepsy
Chalfont Centre for Epilepsy, Chalfont St Peter, Gerrards Cross, Bucks SL9 0RJ

National Society for Mentally Handicapped Children and Adults (MENCAP)
123 Golden Lane, London EC1Y 0RT

National Society for Phenylketonuria and Allied Disorders
B. Tarbot, 26 Towngate Grove, Mirfield, West Yorks WF14 9JT

National Society for the Prevention of Cruelty to Children
1 Riding House Street, London W1P 8AA

National Stillbirth Study Group
66 Harley Street, London W1N 1AE

National Union of Townswomen's Guilds
2 Cromwell Place, London SW7 2JG

Open Door Association
447 Pensby Road, Heswall, Merseyside L61 9PQ

Organization for Parents Under Stress (OPUS)
(many branches offer telephone advice to parents; see local telephone directory)

Parent to Parent Information on Adoption Services
26 Belsize Grove, London NW3 4TR

Parkinsons Disease Society of the United Kingdom
81 Queens Road, London SW19 8NR

Partially Sighted Society
40 Wordsworth Street, Hove, East Sussex BN3 5BH

Patients Association
11 Dartmouth Street, London SW1H 9BN

Phobic Society
4 Cheltenham Road, Chorlton-cum-Hardy, Manchester M21 1QN

Phobic Trust
51 Northwood Avenue, Purley, Surrey CR2 2ER

Physically Handicapped and Able Bodied (PHAB)
42 Devonshire Street, London W1N 1LN
(aims to integrate the physically handicapped into society)

Possum User's Association
14 Greenvale Drive, Timsbury, Bath, Avon BA3 1HP

Pregnancy Advisory Service
40 Margaret Street, London W1N 7FB
(birth control and pregnancy tests; abortions)

Pre-Retirement Association
19 Undine Street, London SW17 8PP

Psoriasis Association
7 Milton Street, Northampton NN2 7JG

Psychiatric Rehabilitation Association
21a Kingsland High Street, London E8 2JS

Rape Crisis Centre
PO Box 42, London N6 5BU (phone (01)340-6913 and (01)340-6145)

Reach – The Association for Children with Artificial Arms
11 Shelley Road, St Marks, Cheltenham, Glos GL51 7LE

Release
1 Elgin Avenue, London W9 3PR
(advice on unwanted pregnancies; will help arrange abortions)

Richmond Fellowship
8 Addison Road, London W14 8DL
(provides support for the mentally and emotionally disturbed)

Riding for the Disabled Association
Avenue R, National Agricultural Centre, Kenilworth, Warwicks CV8 2LY

Royal Association for Disability and Rehabilitation
25 Mortimer Street, London W1N 8AB

Royal National Institute for the Blind
224 Great Portland Street, London W1N 6AA

Royal National Institute for the Deaf
105 Gower Street, London WC1E 6AH

St John Ambulance Association
1 Grosvenor Crescent, London SW1X 7EF
(offers voluntary and practical help for groups and individuals)

Scottish Epilepsy Association
48 Gorvan Road, Glasgow G51 1JL

Salvation Army
PO Box 249, 101 Queen Victoria Street, London EC4P 4EP
(runs many hostels and units for people in need)

Samaritans
17 Uxbridge Road, Slough, Berks SL1 1SN
(offers emergency help and advice to the desperate; has nearly 200 branches;
see local telephone directory for details)

Sappho
The Basement, 20 Dorset Square, London NW1 6QB
(society for lesbians)

Schizophrenia Association of Great Britain
Llanfair Hall, Caernarvon LL55 1TT

SHAFT
4 Adelaide Square, Windsor, Berks SL4 2AQ
(organization which will offer advice to transsexuals)

Shelter (National Campaign for the Homeless)
157 Waterloo Road, London SE1 8XN

Society of Skin Camouflage
Western Pitmenzie, Auchtermuchty, Fife

Society to Support Home Confinements
17 Laburnam Avenue, Durham DH1 4HA

Spastics Society
12 Park Crescent, London W1N 4EQ

Spinal Injuries Association
5 Crowndale Road, London NW1 1TU

Standing Conference on Drug Abuse
3 Blackburn Road, London NW6 1XA

Stillbirth and Perinatal Death Association
51 Christchurch Hill, London NW3 1JY
(organized to help bereaved parents)

Thalidomide Society
19 Upper Hall Park, Berkhamstead, Herts HP4 2NP

Trust Fund for the Training of Handicapped Children in Arts and Crafts
94 Claremount Road, Wallasey, Merseyside L45 6UE

Tuberous Sclerosis Association of Great Britain
Church Farm House, Church Road, North Leigh, Oxford OX8 6TX

Turning Point
8 Strutton Ground, London SW1 2HP
(helps rehabilitate drug addicts and drinkers)

U and I Club (Cystitis)
9e Compton Road, Islington, London N1 2PA

Urinary Conduit Association
36 York Road, Denton, Manchester M34 3HL
(helps all those who have had a urostomy)

Vasectomy
Crediton Project, West Longsight, Crediton, Devon

Voluntary Council for Handicapped Children
8 Wakeley Street, London EC1V 4QE

Volunteer Bone Marrow Register
St Mary Abbots Hospital, Marloes Road, London W8 5LQ

Weight Watchers
635–7 Ajax Avenue, Slough, Berks SL1 4DB

Womens Aid Federation
374 Grays Inn Road, London WC1X 8BB
(support and advice to battered women)

Womens National Cancer Control Campaign
1 South Audley Street, London W1Y 5DQ

Womens Royal Voluntary Service
17 Old Park Lane, London W1Y 4AJ
(runs Meals on Wheels and a hundred other services for those in need)

Investigations
and Tests

A to Z directory of investigations and tests

Any patient who is seen by a doctor will be subjected to a number of investigations. The simplest investigations are those conducted orally — the doctor asks the patient questions and from the answers he receives he will be able to draw specific conclusions. Following the oral examination there will invariably be some sort of physical examination. This may be brief and specific and consist of nothing more than the shining of a torch down the patient's throat, or it may be lengthy and comprehensive and consist of a thorough physical examination in which the practitioner will examine each part of the body in turn. If at this point the diagnosis is still not clear then the doctor, whether he is a GP or a specialist, will want to conduct more exhaustive investigations.

In the sphere of investigations and tests the overlap between GPs and specialists is enormous: there is probably no test done by GPs that is not done by hospital specialists, and possibly no test done by hospital specialists that has not at some time or other been done by a GP. So I have prepared the following single A to Z directory of the most commonly performed investigations. Since reading and studying the results of specific investigations in isolation can be misleading I have deliberately not included figures in this section but have restricted myself to a general discussion of the types of tests most often performed.

amniocentesis
The amniotic fluid is the substance which surrounds the human foetus when it is inside the womb. An examination of this fluid will often tell a doctor a good deal about the baby. Unfortunately, amniocentesis (which involves withdrawing a small portion of the fluid through a needle) is not without risk, and it is only used in a small proportion of pregnancies.

arteriography
X-ray pictures of the interior architecture of arteries can be obtained by injecting them with a substance which will show up on an X-ray and by then taking X-ray photographs (*see* barium meal examination for a more comprehensive explanation of how X-rays work).

audiometry
The measurement of hearing.

barium meal examination
When X-ray photographs are taken only substances which are opaque to X-rays can be seen on the X-ray plate. Bones show up clearly while soft tissues, such as

muscles and fat, hardly show up at all. So radiologists are able to study the shape and condition of particular organs within the body by using an opaque substance such as a barium preparation. For a barium meal examination the patient swallows the barium mixture and the barium goes into the stomach. On the X-ray photograph the barium can be seen clearly and the edges of the barium show where the inside walls of the stomach are. Sometimes the radiologist will actually watch the barium being swallowed and going down into the stomach so that he can see any abnormality which may be present in the gullet or any abnormalities in the swallowing mechanism.

barium enema examination

To get a clear contrast X-ray of the bowel it is necessary to insert the barium mixture directly into the anus. The patient is then tipped up so that the barium flows up the intestinal canal into the colon. Obviously it is important for the patient's bowels to be as empty as possible before this examination is performed and so patients will usually be given a laxative to take before the test is done.

biochemistry

Biochemistry is defined as the study of the chemical reactions which occur within living organisms. A number of the tests done on blood samples are managed by biochemists and technicians working in medical laboratories. Human metabolism is one of the areas covered by the general term 'biochemistry'.

biopsy

A study of living tissue made under a microscope can often reveal more than could be seen with the naked eye when the tissue was still in place. For this reason tissue is sometimes removed from the body and sent along to a pathology laboratory for examination. A wide-bored needle is used for some tests while in others a surgeon simply removes a piece of the tissue he wants examined. Occasionally a surgeon will ask for a biopsy specimen to be examined while the patient remains on the operating table under an anaesthetic. The result of the pathologist's report, which will be telephoned to the operating theatre, may then influence what further surgery is done.

blood tests

It would probably be easier to list the tests which cannot be done on blood samples than to list the tests which can be done! Cells can be examined and the amount of substances such as sugar, alcohol or iron can be estimated accurately. Different tests have to be done on different types of sample (some need to be unclotted, for example) and so when a blood sample has been taken small amounts of the same sample may be placed in different containers.

breast screening

The best way to examine the human breast and exclude the existence of lumps of any kind is still by hand. Women who want to examine their own breasts regularly and who are not sure how to do this should write to the Health Education Council (see p. 169) for an explanatory leaflet or see my book *Aspirin or Ambulance?*

Investigations and Tests

bronchoscopy

The bronchi are the two main tubes which take air down into the lungs. With the aid of a special viewing instrument called a bronchoscope a doctor can see right down into the bronchi and he may even be able to perform small operations inside them.

cardiac catheterization

A heart specialist wanting to know exactly what is going on inside a patient's heart can find out by performing a cardiac catheterization. A thin tube is inserted into a vein, usually in the arm, and then pushed along that vein until it reaches the main chambers of the heart itself. Different pressures in the different parts of the heart can then be measured accurately. In diagnostic terms this is a relatively dangerous investigation which is usually only performed on individuals who have fairly severe or distressing heart symptoms.

cardiac function

When a physician wants to know precisely how well a patient is doing he may not be satisfied with the patient's subjective account of his own progress. If that is the case, he can arrange for the patient to undergo cardiac function tests. The patient may, for example, stand on a moving pavement so that an ordinary walking motion is simulated, with test leads attached to his body. This will enable the physician to study the capacity of the heart directly on an electrocardiogram (*see* electrocardiography).

cervical smears

If a few cells scraped from the cervix (the neck of the womb) are examined under a microscope, a skilled observer may be able to see signs of early malignant changes if any are present. This is obviously, therefore, an extremely important early warning test for cervical cancer. Women who want to have the test done can usually find a screening clinic locally. Many doctors perform the test routinely when examining female patients.

Under present arrangements records of women who have had smears done through NHS clinics are kept at the National Health Service Central Register at Southport so that reminders can be sent out at five-yearly intervals to women living in areas which participate in the central recall scheme. Women living in areas which do not participate in this central scheme may be called through local recording arrangements. Only women over the age of thirty-five (or, if under thirty-five, women who have had three or more pregnancies) are recalled automatically. (These regulations were under review in 1981.)

cholecystography

X-ray pictures showing the gall bladder can be obtained by giving the patient a special substance to swallow. The radio-opaque substance, if it is concentrated within the gall bladder, will be clearly visible on X-ray photographs. Any stones in the gall bladder will then be visible on the resulting X-ray.

colonoscopy

Modern flexible light tubes now enable physicians and surgeons to study much more of the bowel than used to be possible. A few years ago doctors were able only to see those parts of the bowel which could be studied with a rigid tube through which a light could be shone. Today, by using fibreoptic instruments, doctors can study the whole of the large bowel and that includes the whole of the colon.

colposcopy

Invented over half a century ago, the colposcope is used to provide the viewer (usually a gynaecologist) with an illuminated and slightly magnified view of the cervix.

computerized tomography (CT)

Computerized tomography or scanning is expensive and fashionable, and some people think that it has been grossly oversold in recent years. They claim that the many local groups who struggle to raise the money needed to buy and run the extraordinarily complicated equipment involved would do their local hospitals much more good if they spent their time raising money for a new supply of ordinary X-ray equipment.

This is not the place for a full description of how computerized tomography works. It is sufficient to explain that the equipment will enable the specialist radiologist to take what are, effectively, three-dimensional pictures of the part of the body being examined. The camera moves around the body and takes a great many pictures in sequence.

Computerized tomography is undoubtedly a great boon to diagnosticians, but unfortunately in many of the cases successfully diagnosed no treatment is available (because, for example, a lesion discovered is inaccessible).

cystoscopy

If a narrow tube is inserted into the urethra and then pushed as far as the bladder, a viewing urologist can get an excellent sight of the inner walls of the bladder. He can even perform small operations by manipulating delicate instruments which are pushed along the viewing tube.

electrocardiography (ECG)

The electrical activity within a human heart can be measured by attaching leads to the patient's body and then connecting them to a special machine. The machine may enable the viewer to obtain a permanent result (in the form of a thin strip of paper which records the electrical changes in the heart) or a temporary view of what is happening on a small television screen. There is often an accompanying 'beep' to reassure all observers that the heart is beating normally. As all viewers of medical films will know, when the heart stops this beep becomes a continuous sound. A similar result can be obtained by disconnecting the machine, and agitated patients have often been known to alarm nurses and doctors in this way.

electroencephalography (EEG)

The electrical activity within the brain can be measured with a machine called an electroencephalogram. The result of the test appears as many pages of paper on which squiggles denote different types of brain activity. To record the squiggles the patient is connected to the testing machine by a number of wires which, at his end, are attached to his scalp. Shaving of the scalp is not necessary.

endoscopy

This is the generic term used to describe all the '-oscopys' (such as bronchoscopy, laparoscopy and so on). An endoscope is simply a tube which is used to enable the investigator to get a peep inside a part of the human body.

gastroscopy

A gastroscope is an instrument which is pushed down the gullet into the stomach to enable the person using it to study the inside of the stomach directly. Photographs can be taken down the gastroscope and small operations can be performed with its aid. Modern flexible tubes can even be pushed far enough to enable the viewer to study the duodenum.

glucose tolerance test (GTT)

In order to determine whether or not an individual is diabetic it is sometimes necessary to perform a glucose tolerance test. The test is really very simple: the patient is given a large amount of glucose and samples of his blood are tested at intervals afterwards. The rate at which the glucose level in the blood rises and falls helps make the diagnosis.

haematology

This is simply the science of studying the blood and the cells of which the blood is composed. Strictly speaking a haematologist is not interested in substances which may be carried in the blood, such as alcohol or sugar, but in the blood cells themselves.

hormone tests

Measuring the hormone levels within the body is a complex business which is sometimes done with the aid of urine tests and sometimes with the aid of blood tests.

instrument examination

Most doctors use a small number of instruments regularly. The most commonly employed include the following:

    auriscope and otoscope – instruments for looking inside the human ear
    ophthalmoscope – an instrument for examining the inside of the eye
    patella hammer – the small instrument with which doctors elicit reflex reactions
    sphygmomanometer – instrument for measuring blood pressure
    stethoscope – instrument for listening to the heart, chest and abdomen

intravenous pyelography
To obtain a clear picture of the ureters and the bladder and to get a good idea of the effectiveness of the kidneys it is necessary to inject a special dye into the blood stream. X-ray photographs taken afterwards then show the dye being excreted by the kidneys.

laparoscopy *see* peritoneoscopy.

laparotomy
When all investigations have still failed to produce a diagnosis doctors may decide to perform a laparotomy. This simply means that the abdomen will be opened by a surgeon so that he and anyone with him can study the organs within directly.

laryngoscopy
This simple and commonly performed test enables the doctor, using a laryngoscope, to view the larynx and deeper parts of the throat.

lumbar puncture
The brain and the spinal cord are bathed in a fluid called cerebrospinal fluid (known for short as CSF). Testing this fluid sometimes provides valuable diagnostic clues. Unfortunately the sample of fluid needed can only be obtained by inserting a needle into the spine.

lung function
There are several ways in which an examiner can test a patient's lung function. The simplest merely involve the use of instruments which measure the patient's capacity to take in air and to blow it out.

mammography
If special techniques are used soft tissues (such as the breasts) can be pictured with X-ray equipment. Mammography is simply the science of X-raying the breasts.

microscopy
When something is magnified details invisible to the naked eye are revealed. Pathologists may use ordinary magnifying glasses but they also commonly use microscopes of many kinds — varying from the simple light microscope to the more complex and expensive electron microscope which magnifies thousands of times. Blood, urine and tissues of all kinds are subjected to scrutiny under the microscope.

myelography
An X-ray picture of the spinal cord (and of anything pressing on it) can be obtained by injecting a contrasting medium (a substance which is opaque on an X-ray) into the space around the cord.

oesophagoscopy
When the observer wishes only to examine the oesophagus or gullet he can use an oesophagoscope which is a short version of the gastroscope.

Investigations and Tests

pathology
Literally, pathology is simply the study of the changes produced by disease. A pathologist may be experimental (in which case he studies artificially induced changes), comparative (in which case he specializes in comparing human pathology with that of other animals), surgical (which means that he deals mainly with specimens obtained by or for surgeons), forensic (which means that he specializes in disease and death associated with crime), or general. Pathologists are medically qualified and their laboratories usually have the responsibility for organizing blood, urine and swab tests of many kinds as well as coordinating most of the tests done on tissue samples.

peak flow meter
A hundred years ago doctors who wanted to test the respiratory efficiency of their patients would ask them to try and blow out a candle. The peak flow meter was designed to put this test on to a scientific basis. The patient simply blows through a mouthpiece on to a spring-loaded trigger. The trigger moves a pointer on a scale. The value of this instrument is that it enables the doctor to measure rates of deterioration or improvement and thereby to judge accurately the effectiveness of treatments he tries.

peritoneoscopy
The peritoneum is the membranous lining inside the abdominal walls and covering the intestines and a peritoneoscope is an instrument which, when pushed through an incision made in the abdominal wall enables an investigator to study the peritoneum. There is no real difference between peritoneoscopy and laparoscopy as far as the patient is concerned.

proctoscopy
The proctoscope is the shortest of the tubes used for examining the large bowel and it enables the viewer to see those few inches of the rectum which are just outside the reach of the examining finger.

radioactive isotopes test
A radioactive isotope of iodine is sometimes used in the examination of the thyroid gland. The rate at which the radioactive iodine is taken up by the gland is increased in thyrotoxidosis.

scanning
see computerized tomography.

sigmoidoscopy
The lower or more distal part of the colon is known as the sigmoid colon, and the long metal instrument which enables the surgeon or physician to study that part of the bowel is known as a sigmoidoscope. The instrument is pushed gently inside the rectum and through it the observer can study the walls of the colon and even take biopsy samples.

swab tests

When a sample of material from a wound or from any other site is tested and investigated it is usually possible to identify any organisms present and to get a good idea of drugs which may prove effective against them. In dictionary terms a 'swab' is a small piece of cotton wrapped around a slender wooden stick. The sample is obtained by wiping the swab across the surface to be studied.

test meal

In order to test the functioning of the intestinal tract doctors sometimes give patients a test meal which consists, just as the name suggests, of a carefully prepared portion of food.

thermography

The human body permanently emits infra-red radiation and with the aid of expensive, sensitive equipment the amount of radiation can be accurately measured. The colourful and rather exotic thermograms which can be obtained in this way help to provide a picture of the physiological and pathological processes going on inside the body.

ultrasound

Ultrasonic vibrations are high-frequency sound waves which are inaudible to the human ear and are capable of travelling through the soft tissues of the body at a constant speed. The vibrations are deflected when they reach the boundaries between structures of a different density and it is this fact which makes them such a valuable addition to the diagnostician's armoury. Ultrasonic vibrations are widely used in obstetrics to help obstetricians confirm pregnancy, check when they think that there is a possibility of a multiple pregnancy and locate the position and development of the foetus. There is believed to be much less risk to mother and foetus when ultrasound is used than when ordinary X-rays are used.

urine tests

Modern technology has simplified urine testing a great deal. A few years ago,doctors wishing to examine the contents of a urine specimen would have to conduct complex, lengthy and time consuming experiments. Today they can do a number of simple tests with small strips of specially prepared paper or with the aid of small specially constituted tablets. These strips and tablets enable doctors to test for protein, sugar, blood and bilirubin among other things. When an infection is suspected, however, the sample needs to be examined under a microscope and the sensitivity of any infective material to the various available drugs has to be assessed on special culture plates. Some GPs perform their own microscopic urine examinations but most send off specimens to the local pathology laboratory. Incidentally, if a specimen is to be tested for infection then two important requirements must be met. First, the specimen must be a 'mid-stream' one – that means that it is not the first spurt of urine to appear from the urethra nor the last. Second, the specimen must be placed in a special sterile bottle and not in any old whisky or herb jar.

Testing urine for signs of pregnancy is sometimes done by GPs but again this is usually something done in the local hospital laboratory. There are in addition, however, a number of commercial laboratories which do pregnancy testing, and there are useful home-testing kits available which are said to be extremely reliable if used according to the manufacturer's instructions.

venography
If contrast material is injected into veins X-ray pictures can be taken.

ventriculography
If air is injected into the ventricles or spaces within the brain X-ray photographs will enable a skilled observer to study the anatomy of the brain in some detail. This procedure is also known as air encephalography.

xerography
This technique uses ordinary X-rays and a process said to be similar to the one used to reproduce documents. The technique requires an increased dose of X-rays and is therefore not widely used at the moment. It is used to photograph the breasts.

X-rays
Discovered accidentally by an observant physicist called Roentgen at the end of the 19th century, X-rays have helped to revolutionize medical care throughout the world. With the aid of X-rays doctors can study not only the human skeleton but also the organs and tissues within the body. It is true that only bones show up clearly when an X-ray is taken of an ordinary naked body but by using opaque substances (as in a barium meal) the internal organs can also be displayed clearly.

Drugs and Treatments

- [ ] *Prescription Drugs*
- [ ] *Operative Procedures*
- [ ] *Other Forms of Treatment*
- [ ] *Home Care*

☐ Prescription Drugs

There are very many aspects of drug production, testing and marketing which are rightly subjects of public concern, but here I have confined myself to a brief study of those topics which are of direct interest to the consumer of medical care and medicinal products.

Obtaining a 'prescription only' drug

Registered medical practitioners alone are entitled to sign prescriptions for drugs on the 'prescription only' list.

A registered practitioner may work in hospital or general practice and he may provide a health service prescription or a private prescription. The prescription, when written and signed, may be dispensed by a hospital or community pharmacist or by the doctor himself.

When cashing a health service prescription at a community pharmacy a patient will have to pay the standard prescription charge unless he has an exemption certificate. When cashing a private prescription a patient must pay the price of the drug concerned plus the pharmacist's handling charge. Private prescriptions usually cost more than the standard NHS prescription fee.

All GPs are legally obliged to provide drugs needed in an emergency and they may claim payment for supplying drugs to patients if the patients would have difficulty in obtaining the products or if there are no chemists' shops within one mile. Private patients can be supplied by GPs with whatever drugs they need. The doctor is responsible for making any appropriate charge.

A patient who runs out of a medicine needed regularly and who is not able to obtain a prescription may obtain an emergency three-day supply from a pharmacist (or a five-day supply if the three days include a public holiday) as long as the drug is not on a controlled list and the pharmacist is persuaded that the need is genuine.

Categories of prescription drugs

There are many laws controlling the sale and purchase of drugs but the simplest dividing line is the one separating the drugs which can be purchased freely over the counter without a doctor's prescription and the drugs which can only be obtained with a prescription. In legal terms, of course, the products which fall into the first category, and can be bought freely, also fall into the second category, and may be prescribed by registered medical practitioners.

The group of drugs that can only be obtained with a doctor's prescription is further divided and those particularly dangerous products (such as the powerful pain killers) are subject to stringent controls and have to be prescribed and dispensed with particular care. The regulations which govern the control of these particularly powerful drugs are of little practical concern to consumers apart from the fact that prescriptions must be written out in a particular way.

Prescriptions for controlled drugs must be in ink or otherwise indelible, must be signed by the doctor concerned and dated by him, and the name and address of the patient together with the details of the drug itself must all be in the doctor's own handwriting. The details of the drug on the prescription must include the strength, the form, and the number of tablets or phials to be prescribed. The number of tablets or phials must be written in words as well as figures. The dose must also be written on the prescription in the doctor's own handwriting. The chemist will not supply a controlled drug if these conditions are not met.

197

The variety of products available

Although the World Health Organization has estimated that few prescribers need more than 200 drugs in their armamentarium there are many thousands of drug products on the market. There are considerably more than 20,000 drugs available in Britain.

A great many of these products are virtually identical in chemical value. There are, for example, scores of indigestion remedies containing the same basic ingredients, dozens of antibiotics with similar properties, and a great many pain killers, contraceptive pills, sleeping tablets and tranquillizers. Doctors choosing which product to prescribe have much the same sort of problem as customers in a chemist's shop trying to decide which headache remedy to choose.

The number of genuinely different, 'new' drugs introduced onto the market each year is very small. The number of alternative drugs introduced is enormous.

Branded or generic?

Every drug that a doctor prescribes will fall into one of two groups: branded and generic. The term generic simply means that the name is a general one describing a type of pharmacological product and is not associated with any particular manufacturer. The name 'tetracycline' is, for example, a generic name and a large number of manufacturers produce drugs which can be described as 'tetracycline'. The name Imperacin, however, is a brand name given by Imperial Chemical Industries (ICI) to a particular tetracycline product.

In practice, if a doctor writes a prescription for Imperacin then the chemist must dispense tablets of tetracycline made by ICI. If the doctor writes a prescription for tetracycline the chemist may dispense tablets of tetracycline made by any manufacturer.

Doctors obtain a great deal of their prescribing information from drug manufacturers who obviously describe drugs by their brand name. It would hardly be appropriate for ICI to extol the virtues of all tetracycline products any more than it would for the Ford Motor Car Company to extol the virtues of, say, estate cars in general.

Because their information comes from this biased source, and because the drug companies usually manage to give their products names that are shorter and easier to remember than the generic names handed out by manufacturing chemists and official committees, most doctors prescribe branded products rather than generic products. The drug companies claim that this is wise because branded products are made according to strict regulations. Spokesmen for the DHSS, on the other hand, argue that branded products are nearly always more expensive than generic products and that the regulations governing the manufacturer of generic products are strict enough to ensure that there is little practical difference between a generic product and a branded product.

Drug efficiency

Drug companies only have to provide evidence that their drugs are safe before they can obtain marketing licences; they do not have to produce any evidence that they work.

Inevitably this means that a large number of inefficient, ineffective drugs are available on prescription. Many of these drugs rely on the 'placebo effect' (see p. 200) for any value they may have.

Among the drugs most commonly described as ineffective and not worth prescribing are many of the combination remedies which contain two or more individual drugs in one compound. The 1981 *British National Formulary*, published jointly by the British Medical Association and the Pharmaceutical Society of Great Britain, lists 600 drugs which are described as 'less suitable for prescribing' than other medicines.

Patients' expectations

A number of surveys have shown that a large percentage of patients feel cheated if they leave the doctor's surgery without a prescription. It has been said that to some patients a visit to the doctor's surgery that does not end in the handing over of a prescription is as disappointing as a child's visit to Father Christmas's Grotto which does not end up with the handing over of a present.

Many doctors undoubtedly subscribe to this rather patronizing viewpoint and encourage the perpetuation of the myth by ending all their consultations with a scrawl on a prescription pad.

Patients who are prepared to leave the surgery without a prescription should perhaps make this point as tactfully as possible at some point during their consultation.

It does, incidentally, now look as though doctors are too willing to prescribe and patients know better. An American survey has shown that 80 per cent of Americans feel that doctors are too quick to prescribe and 60 per cent feel that some old-fashioned remedies are more effective than the newer products favoured by doctors.

Placebos

Approximately one-third of all patients will obtain relief from tablets and medicines which contain absolutely no pharmacologically active constituents and which work by intent rather than by any immediately discernible physiological effect.

Even patients suffering from severe pain have benefited from the so-called placebo effect and dozens of reliable studies have shown that patients suffering genuine discomfort have obtained noticeable relief from the use of sugar tablets.

Recent research has shown that when a placebo is taken with good effect a special hormone seems to be released by the brain.

This hormone is part of the body's own internal defence mechanism and it seems likely that the placebo pill is simply triggering an automatic release of a pain-relieving product. Since placebos only work when the patient believes that they will work the placebo effect is more marked among anxious, rather dependent individuals than among strong-willed, self-sufficient, suspicious people.

Those who oppose the use of placebos claim that to deceive the patient is wrong even if he benefits and that there is a real risk of turning a healthy patient into a hypochondriac by giving him a placebo.

Those who favour the use of placebos claim that even some of our most pharmacologically effective drugs frequently do their job because of the placebo reaction, and that, whether doctors and patients recognize it or not, between a third and a half of all prescriptions are given partly or wholly for their placebo effect.

How drugs should be taken

It is a sad but true fact that of all the drugs prescribed only a relatively small number are taken in the way that the prescriber originally intended them to be taken. Drugs are taken at the wrong time, they are taken with food when they should be taken before food, they are forgotten, they are taken too frequently and they are sometimes never taken out of the bottle at all.

It is important to remember that modern prescribed drugs are not only potentially effective but also powerful and potentially dangerous. Drug companies spend a considerable amount of money on refining their manufacturing processes and on ensuring that the drugs they make will be made available to the appropriate tissues within the body at a suitable rate. Taking pills at the wrong time or in the wrong way can devalue such careful preparation.

There are several questions which should be answered before a patient starts taking a drug. Usually the answers to these questions will appear on the label of the bottle containing the drugs. If the answers do not appear there then the fault may lie with the doctor who wrote the prescription or the pharmacist who dispensed it.

For how long must the drug be taken and in what dosage?

Some drugs can be stopped when symptoms cease. Others need to be taken as a complete course. A small number of drugs need to be taken continuously and a second prescription will have to be obtained when the first supply has run out. The patient who knows what his drug is for, why he is taking it and what the effect should be, will be more likely to know when a drug is to be stopped. The alphabetical list on pp. 225–67 is designed to facilitate understanding.

How many times a day must the drug be taken?

If a drug has to be taken once a day, it does not usually matter what time of day it is taken, as long as it is taken at the same time each day. If a drug has to be taken twice a day it should be taken at intervals of 12 hours. A drug that needs taking three times a day should be taken at eight-hourly intervals and a drug that needs taking four times a day should be taken at six-hourly intervals. The day should be divided into suitable segments.

Does it matter whether the drug is taken before meals, during meals or after meals?

Some drugs which may cause stomach problems are safer when taken with meals. Other drugs may not be absorbed properly if taken with food.

If a new drug is being added to a collection of other pills being taken regularly how can mistakes be avoided?

A number of patients (particularly the elderly) are expected to remember to take dozens of pills a day. When a day's medication includes tablets to be taken twice daily, three times daily, mornings only and every four hours, mistakes are inevitable.

If a patient needs to take a number of drugs a day mistakes can be minimized by preparing a daily chart on which the names and times of different drugs are marked. Such a chart will reduce the risk of a patient taking one dose twice or struggling to remember whether a particular pill has been taken yet. Two commercial drug boxes, which contain small compartments in which each day's drugs can be placed, are available. These are Dosett, marketed by Penmill Ltd, 20 Ivy Bank Park, Entry Hill, Bath BA2 5NF, and Medidos, made by Pharmagen Ltd, Chapel Street, Runcorn, Cheshire WA7 5AP.

Overdosage

To avoid the risk of overdosage sleeping tablets should not be kept by the bedside. It is too easy for a half-asleep patient to mistakenly take extra tablets. In the case of a suspected overdose medical attention must be sought (see p. 214).

Drug route

Traditionally most drugs are taken by mouth or given by injection.

In recent years, however, the popularity of other types of presentation has increased. For example, an increasing number of patients now take their drugs in suppository form. This has for many years been an accepted route in France. The main advantage is that stomach upsets are completely avoided.

Even more recently there has been a dramatic increase in the interest shown in products designed to be used through the skin. There are now products available as creams and ointments designed to have an effect on the whole body. Hormones, for example, seem particularly suitable for this type of preparation.

It seems very likely that in the future a considerable amount of research will be done on drug presentation as well as drug content. Patients should, perhaps, be prepared to receive prescriptions for drugs designed to be used in rather unusual ways.

Storing medicines

Medicines should be stored in the containers in which they were supplied and the labels should not be removed. Containers should be kept tightly fastened and out of extremes of both heat and cold. If there is an expiry date on a prescription medicine then the medicine should either be returned to the chemist or emptied down the lavatory on or after that date.

Any prescribed medicines not needed on a regular basis should be thrown away without delay while any prescribed medicines which are taken regularly should be thrown away after six months if there is no earlier expiry date. Any medicine that changes in appearance should be discarded (see also p. 307).

To pay or not to pay

All health service patients obtaining prescriptions from family doctors must pay the standard prescription fee unless they are in one of the exempt categories. There are several such categories.

1 Children under sixteen

2 Men aged sixty-five and over

3 Women aged sixty and over

4 Expectant mothers who have Family Practitioner Committee exemption certificates

5 Mothers with one or more children under one year old

6 Patients receiving supplementary benefit or family income supplement and any other patients who hold DHSS exemption certificates

7 War and service pensioners who require prescriptions for products to treat the disability which merits the pension.

8 Patients suffering from the following complaints: a permanent fistula, such as a colostomy; diabetes mellitus (sugar diabetes); myxoedema; epilepsy; myasthenia gravis; hypoadrenalism (Addison's disease); hypopituitarism; any continuing physical disability which prevents the patient from leaving home without assistance

9 Patients who have a pre-payment certificate (FP96) bought from the local Family Practitioner Committee (with an application on form FP95)

An application for a prescription charge exemption certificate should be made on form FP91.

Patients who consider that they may be exempt but who do not have the appropriate certificate of exemption should ask for a receipt on form FP57. With the aid of this form they can obtain a refund if they are entitled to one.

Repeat prescriptions

By no means all the prescriptions signed by GPs are the result of specific requests for diagnostic aid and therapeutic intervention. A growing number of prescriptions (now said to be about half of all those written) are provided without there being any meeting between the doctor and the patient. The patient writes or telephones for a new supply of a specific drug and then, a day or so later, either collects or receives through the post the appropriate prescription.

This system of providing prescriptions 'on request' was originally designed to help patients suffering from chronic disorders such as diabetes, high blood pressure or epilepsy. Patients suffering from disorders which tend to vary very little over the months do not need regular medical examinations but they do

205

need regular supplies of drugs. For them to have to visit a doctor simply to obtain a prescription is a waste of everyone's time. Doctors do not usually prescribe quantities of drugs likely to last more than four to six weeks since some drugs deteriorate if kept too long and most practitioners feel that it is unwise to allow any patient to keep excessively large quantities of drugs at home.

Unfortunately, repeat prescribing is not always restricted to patients with long-term problems requiring continuous medication. Patients who really should see a doctor rather than continue taking tablets sometimes ask for repeat prescriptions and, to the shame of the medical profession, not infrequently obtain them. Many patients have become psychologically dependent upon sleeping tablets and tranquillizers because of the ease with which they have been able to obtain repeat prescriptions.

Arrangements for obtaining repeat prescriptions vary a good deal from practice to practice. In some practices patients entitled to receive prescriptions are issued with cards on which the drugs which they are allowed to receive without any consultation are listed. There may be a limit on the number of prescriptions which any patient may obtain without being reviewed. In other practices the cards detailing drugs which can be provided on repeat prescriptions are kept with the patient's notes so that the receptionists, who usually write out repeat prescriptions, can check on drugs, and dosages, and make a note of the number of prescriptions issued.

Theoretically, doctors signing prescriptions should check all the details, including specific points such as the dosages and quantities of drugs to be supplied, and general points such as the suitability of continuing with the treatment. In practice many prescriptions supplied in this way are signed almost without the doctor looking at them.

For this reason I suggest that patients receiving drugs on repeat prescriptions should always check that the tablets they receive match the tablets previously prescribed and that any instructions on the bottle label match previous instructions. If there is any

The top ten prescription groups

1 Drugs acting on the nervous system, including sleeping tablets, pain killers, anti-anxiety pills

2 Anti-infectives such as penicillin

3 Respiratory tract drugs, including cough medicines

4 Heart drugs

5 Drugs acting on the alimentary tract, including laxatives and indigestion remedies

6 Skin preparations

7 Nutrition and blood preparations, including iron and vitamin products

8 Ear, nose and eye preparations

9 Rheumatic disease products

10 Drugs acting on metabolism, including hormones

This list refers to therapeutic drugs; the contraceptive pill would otherwise figure prominently

confusion or uncertainty then a telephone call should be made to the surgery and the tablets should not be used.

As a general rule, I suggest that only patients who have established and long-term clinical problems should obtain drugs on repeat prescriptions and they should visit the surgery at least once every six months to check that the medication does not need changing. Patients with short-term or acute conditions who need medication should always speak to a doctor.

Drugs during pregnancy

No pregnant woman should take any drug or medicine unless it has been prescribed for her by a doctor who knows that she is pregnant. This means that a woman on long-term medication who becomes pregnant must revisit her doctor, that no woman should take a drug prescribed by a doctor who may not be aware that she is pregnant and that no pregnant woman should take any home medicine without permission from her doctor.

A statement issued by the Committee on Safety of Medicines in February 1981 concluded that 'it is impossible to prove beyond a shadow of a doubt that any drug is absolutely safe in pregnancy' and that 'drugs should not be given during pregnancy unless they are essential'.

Incidentally, some particularly cautious doctors assume that all women of child-bearing age are pregnant until proved otherwise and may refuse to prescribe until assured on this point.

Drugs during breastfeeding

The increase in the number of women breastfeeding their babies is matched by the increase in the number of different drugs taken by new mothers. Although some drugs may well have no effect on the newborn baby and may not be excreted in the breast milk I believe that caution is sensible. The amount of evidence on this subject is still very slight.

In general, I would recommend that no mother should breast-feed while taking a drug unless assured by her own GP or by the doctor looking after her that it is safe for her to do so.

Drugs for children

Children are not just miniature adults, and they do not always metabolize drugs in the same way that adults do. This means that the popular practice of simply reducing the adult dose of a drug when prescribing it for a child is not a particularly sensible one. Unfortunately, many of the drugs available today have not been effectively tested on children, and there is often no information available to enable practitioners to judge precisely how and what to prescribe.

It is, for this reason, particularly important to ensure that children are only given drugs when no alternative form of treatment is available.

Some children have difficulty in swallowing tablets or capsules and this problem can occasionally be overcome by hiding the tablets in small quantities of a favourite food offered on a tea-spoon. Tablets should not be crushed and capsules should not be opened before being taken since such action may affect the safety and effectiveness of the product.

When liquids are prescribed it is important to shake the bottle before pouring out the recommended dose, since some liquid preparations may separate during storage. Small children who refuse to take medicine can be encouraged to cooperate if the adult giving the medicine holds the child's nose gently but firmly shut and then slips the spoonful of medicine into the mouth. The swallowing reflex will do the rest.

Medicine intended for children should be stored with the same degree of caution as medicine intended for adults.

Unwanted effects of drugs

Side effects caused by drugs are common. One survey has shown that over 40 per cent of all patients receiving drugs suffer a reaction of one kind or another to the drug prescribed. Some of the effects are temporary and fairly minor and cause a minimum of inconvenience, while others are permanent and dangerous. A small number of patients taking prescription drugs die as a result of the drug they have taken. Certain side effects are commoner with specific types and groups of drugs and I offer the following list as a general guide.

Drowsiness

This is a common problem with all drugs which have an effect on the central nervous system – these include sedatives, tranquillizers, hypnotics, all drugs used in the treatment of anxiety and depression and drugs used in the treatment of epilepsy. Drowsiness is also common with antihistamines – the group of drugs used in the treatment of a wide range of allergy problems. Patients taking medication for hay fever should, for example, beware of this problem. Because of the risk of drowsiness patients taking new forms of medication should be particularly careful when driving or operating machinery of any kind. When possible it is wise to begin taking such products at the weekend when contact with machinery can be kept to a minimum.

Nausea and vomiting

A very wide range of drugs can cause nausea and sickness. Hormones, heart drugs, pain relievers and anti-infectives are four of the common groups associated with these side effects.

Dizziness

Aspirin and quinine are two drugs commonly and specifically associated with dizziness. Anti-infectives, blood pressure reducing drugs (hypotensives) and drugs used in the treatment of nerve disorders (such as anxiety and depression) are also common culprits.

Diarrhoea

Anti-infectives (such as types of penicillin) are often associated with diarrhoea as are drugs used in the treatment of gastro-intestinal problems such as indigestion, gastritis and constipation.

Headache

Headache is a symptom that has been associated with an enormous range of drugs. It is, however, important to remember that anxiety and tension are also common causes of headache and that an individual ill enough to need medication may already be anxious or tense.

Dry mouth

Drugs used in the treatment of high blood pressure and/or in the treatment of nervous problems can produce a dry mouth. So can a number of other products.

Indigestion or wind

Obviously drugs that are taken by mouth are most likely to be associated with indigestion and wind. Pain relievers, anti-infectives and steroids are particularly likely to cause these symptoms.

Skin rash

Any drug can cause this side effect. Anti-infectives, such as penicillin and sulphonamide, are perhaps most commonly associated with the problem. A skin rash usually suggests an allergy to the drug (see p. 213).

Itching

Itching associated with a skin rash means that an allergy reaction is almost certain (see 'Skin rash', and p. 213).

Constipation

Common with pain relievers, antacids, cough medicines and, naturally enough, drugs used in the treatment of diarrhoea.

Other effects

Other effects which may commonly be noticed include confusion, hallucination, tremors, fainting, wheezing, palpitations, blurred vision, hot flushes, depression, sweating, ringing in the ears, frigidity and impotence.

What to do when you notice a side effect

The importance of a side effect will obviously vary enormously from symptom to symptom and from individual to individual. There are no specific rules which can safely guide patients suffering from side effects, but in general I would suggest that when side effects are troublesome or persistent medical advice should be sought. Mildly irritating side effects (slight constipation for example) can usually be safely ignored.

When side effects are troublesome or persistent it is usually wiser to contact the doctor rather than simply to stop the treatment. On some occasions stopping the treatment may be potentially more dangerous than coping with the side effects. On other occasions drug treatment may need to be stopped slowly and in careful stages.

If in doubt it is always wise to ask, and a telephone enquiry to your doctor need not take more than a few moments.

What the doctor should do when he is told of a side effect

All doctors are encouraged to make reports to the Committee on Safety of Medicines if they believe that any product they have prescribed has been responsible for an adverse reaction of any kind. Doctors can obtain special postage-paid cards on which to make such reports, but the CSM itself estimates that no more than 10 per cent of all serious drug reactions are reported.

The director of one specialist drug surveillance unit has estimated that there are seven main reasons why GPs do not report adverse reactions. These are:

an ambition to collect together a number of reactions so that a career-boosting research paper can be prepared and published

a belief that all drugs on the market are safe enough

a feeling of guilt at having prescribed a product that might have caused a bad reaction

a fear of being sued if the drug is shown to be responsible for the side effect

an ignorance of the reporting procedure

diffidence

laziness

The Committee on Safety of Medicines can be reached at Market Towers, 1 Nine Elms Lane, London SW8 5NQ.

Sensitivity reactions

Some patients cannot take some drugs without coming out in a red, itchy rash and developing other signs of sensitivity. Penicillin is one of the drugs most commonly associated with this type of allergy reaction.

Once a patient has shown unequivocal signs of a drug allergy care should be taken not to expose the patient to that drug again. A second reaction may be more serious.

The patient's doctor will normally make a note on the medical records but it may also be wise to invest in a Medic Alert bracelet (see p. 337).

Drug interactions

Many drugs do not mix well together and may indeed react together in a dangerous way. Since a large number of patients regularly take two or more drugs this is a real problem. Patients already taking prescribed drugs who are offered prescriptions for additional products should ask their doctor to confirm that the drugs will not interact badly. Patients taking prescribed drugs should not take drugs bought over the counter.

Boehringer Ingelheim publish a 'Drug interaction chart' which lists a wide variety of ways in which drugs may interact badly. The chart is available from the company (address p. 286) to members of the medical and allied professions.

Misuse of drugs

Remarkably many drugs have been misused at one time or another. The greatest problems of addiction and dependence do not, however, involve obvious junkies but respectable individuals hooked on barbiturates, benzodiazepines and other drugs with a stimulant, sedative or tranquillizing effect. The differences between habituation, addiction and dependence are largely theoretical and the dividing line between psychological dependence and physiological dependence is often a thin one.

Poisoning

Anyone suspected of having taken an accidental or deliberate overdose of any drug needs medical attention. Either telephone your own GP or arrange for the patient to be taken immediately to the nearest casualty department.

Any container with or without remaining drugs should be taken with the patient.

A 24-hour Poisons Information Service has centres in Belfast, Cardiff, Dublin, Edinburgh and London. The Service exists to provide doctors with information designed to facilitate treatment of victims of poisoning.

The telephone numbers of the National Poisons Information Service are as follows:

Belfast	0232 30503
Cardiff	0222 492233
Dublin	0001 745588
Edinburgh	031–229 2477
London	01-407 7600

Tips for getting the best out of prescribed drugs

1 Follow any specific instructions that you are given.

2 Learn the names and purposes of the drugs you take. If you are not sure when to take the drugs that you have been given ask your doctor or the pharmacist. If you think you will forget the instructions you are given ask for them to be written down. If you want to know more about the drugs you are taking see the drugs table on pp. 225–67 and the reference books listed on pp. 339–40. The name of the drug you are taking should always appear on the container.

3 Do not remaove drugs from their proper containers except when you need them or if you are transferring them to a device intended to improve compliance (see p. 203).

4 It is wise to assume that until proved otherwise all prescribed drugs can cause drowsiness. If after taking a drug for three days there is no sign of any drowsiness then the problem is unlikely to appear.

5 Drugs do not mix well with alcohol. If you intend to drink and take drugs then ask your doctor whether or not it will be safe. If you are taking more than one prescribed drug it is wise to check with your doctor that the combination is safe. Do not take non-prescribed medicine while taking prescribed medication. Some foods are dangerous with certain drugs and if you are warned not to eat certain foods then take care to follow the advice.

6 Store drugs in a locked cupboard where the temperature is fairly stable.

7 Never take drugs prescribed for someone else. Discard all unused supplies of prescribed drugs. They can either be returned to the chemist or flushed down the lavatory.

8 Do not stop taking drugs suddenly if you have been advised to take a full course. Ring your doctor for advice if you need to stop for any reason. Some drugs have to be stopped gradually rather than abruptly.

9 Try to see the same doctor as often as possible. If several doctors are prescribing for you there is an increased risk of an interaction between drugs which do not mix well.

10 Be on the look-out for side effects, and remember that if you seem to develop a second illness the chances are high that it was caused by the treatment for the first. Some of the commonest side effects are listed on pp. 210ff., but it is important to realize that the side effects commonly associated with specific drugs are only the ones that have been reported, and the Committee on Safety of Medicines estimates that only one in ten drug reactions are reported. So if the side effect you suffer has not been recorded before, don't assume that it is not caused by the drug you are taking.

11 Use drugs with care and caution, but do use them when they are required. Doctors sometimes divide patients into two main groups: those who are willing to take drugs for any little symptom and who feel deprived if not offered a pharmacological solution to every ailment, and those who are unwilling to take drugs under any circumstances. Try not to fall into either of these extremist groups.

Reading a prescription

Hospital patients do not usually see a prescription: if they are in-patients they will usually be given their medication directly by a nurse; if they are out-patients they will simply be given a supply by a representative of the hospital pharmacist.

On the other hand, patients who visit GPs who do not themselves dispense will have to take a prescription form to a local pharmacist. The form used is known as FP10 (see p. 67) and to the majority of patients it will be quite incomprehensible.

In fact, it is quite easy to learn to 'read' a prescription. Patients who learn how to do this will be able to check that the medication the pharmacist supplies matches the doctor's instructions.

In memory of a classical training that few of them have had doctors usually write many of their instructions in Latin using abbreviations that would not always satisfy strict grammarians. A list of the most commonly used abbreviations appears on pp. 220–21. The language that doctors use is often described as 'dog Latin' to distinguish it from more accurate, formal versions of that dead language.

A sample prescription form with guiding notes is included overleaf.

A sample prescription form

1   This part of the form is often left blank. The idea is to avoid the wasting of medicine by allowing the doctor to prescribe the exact quantity that will be required. If the doctor decides that seven days' treatment is necessary and that the patient must take four tablets a day he simply writes '7' in this box. This saves him the task of multiplying 7 by 4 and writing down the total (as in note 5). Obviously where two or more items are included on one prescription (as here) this part of the form may be inappropriate.

2   The letters 'NP' here stand for the Latin for 'proper name'. If this part of the form is left blank the chemist will write the name of the drug prescribed on the bottle, whereas a cross here keeps the name off the bottle.

3   Ampicillin is a generic drug used in the treatment of infections. The letter 'C' is used to tell the pharmacist that the drug should be dispensed in capsule form. The numbers after the name of the drug tell the pharmacist the strength of each individual dose – in this case the size of each dose should be 250 mg.

4   The 'i' suggests that one capsule at a time should be taken and the 'qds' is an abbreviation referring to a Latin phrase which means 'four times a day'.

5   This is the total number of capsules that should be dispensed. The doctor wants his patient to take four capsules a day and has obviously decided on a seven-day course – hence the total of twenty-eight capsules.

6   Mogadon is a brand-name sleeping tablet. The letter 'T' tells the pharmacist to dispense the drug in tablet form.

7   The 'ii' means that two tablets should be taken as a single dose, and the letters 'on' represent the Latin phrase for 'at night'. The pharmacist should, therefore, write instructions on the bottle telling the patient to take two tablets at night.

8   This is the number of tablets that the doctor wants dispensed, so the tablets will last for fifteen days. General practitioners frequently prescribe drugs for a month at a time.

9   The letter 'M' is an abbreviation that means that the drug is to be prescribed as a medicine in liquid form. 'Gent Alk' is a shortened form of gentian alkali and the letters 'BPC' tell the pharmacist that the product should be prepared according to the formulation listed in the British Pharmaceutical Codex.

10   The dose recommended is 10 ml and the prescriber has ordered the medicine to be taken 'tds', or three times a day.

11   The letters 'ac' tell the pharmacist to add 'before meals' to the instructions on the bottle label.

12   The total amount of medicine dispensed is to be 300 ml. This is a common, standard size for liquid medicines and, at 10 ml a time three times a day, will provide enough medicine for ten days.

Remember that different doctors prepare prescriptions in different ways. Not all practitioners use dog Latin abbreviations, for example.

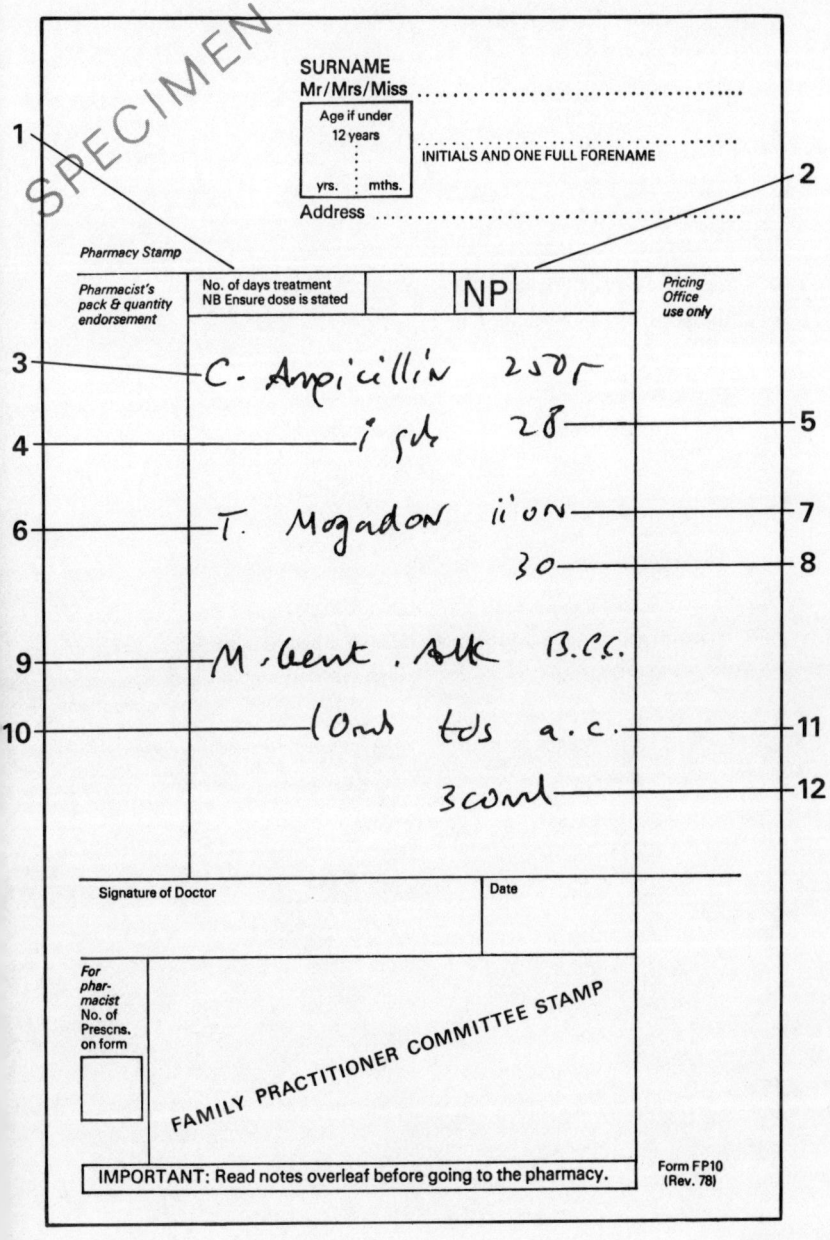

A dog Latin dictionary

ABBREVIATION	LATIN	ENGLISH
aa	ana	of each
ac	ante cibum	before meals
ad lib	ad libitum	freely
alt die	alt diebus	alternate days
alt noct	alt noctibus	alternate nights
aqua calida	aqua calida	hot water
bal	balneum	bath
bd	bis in die	twice a day
bid	bis in die	twice a day
c	cum	with
cat	cataplasma	a poultice
cc	cum	with
cm	cras mane	tomorrow morning
cn	cras nocte	tomorrow evening
dol urg	dolore urgente	when the pain is severe
eq	equalis	equal
ex aq	ex aqua	in water
ext	extractum	extract
f	fiat	let it be made
flav	flavus	yellow
fol	folium	leaf
fs	semi	half
ft	fiat	let it be made
gutt	guttae	drops
haust	haustus	draught
hn	hac nocte	tonight
hor decub	hora decubitus	at bedtime
hs	hora somni	at bedtime
m	misce	mix
m et sign	misce et signa	mix and label
m ft mist	misce fiat mistura	mix and let a mixture be made

md	more dicto	as directed
mdu	more dicto utendus	to be used as directed
mist	mistura	mixture
mit	mitte	send
om	omni mane	every morning
on	omni nocte	every evening
paa	parti effecti applicandus	to be applied to the affected part
p oc	pro oculis	for the eyes
prn	pro re nata	when needed
pulv	pulvis	powder
qd	quater in die	four times a day
qh	quatis horis	four hourly
qid	quater in die	four times a day
qq	quaque	every
qqh	quarta quaque hora	every fourth hour
qs	quantum sufficiat	as much as is sufficient
r	recipe	take thou
rep	repetatur	let it be repeated
rep dos	repetatur dosis	let the dose be repeated
si dol urg	si dolor urgeat	if the pain is severe
sig	signetur	let it be labelled
sig	signa	label
sos	si opus sit	if necessary
ss	semi	half
stat	statim	immediately
syr	syrupus	syrup
td	ter in die	three times a day
tds	ter die sumendum	three times a day
tert qq hora	tertia quaque hora	every third hour
tid	ter in die	three times a day
ung	unguentum	ointment
ut dict	ut dictum	as directed

A to Z of commonly prescribed drugs

On the following pages are listed brief details of several hundred of the most commonly prescribed drugs, including both branded and generic (see p. 198) products. I have resisted the temptation to offer critical, subjective assessments of particular drugs. I have strong views about the suitability of certain drugs for general sale but I do not think that this is the right place to parade those views. The purpose of the following table is to enable readers to learn a little about the drugs they are taking. The suitability of specific drugs in particular circumstances must be a question to be considered by the prescribing physician who is the only person with access to all the relevant information.

I have assumed that the patient who wishes to find out more about the drug he or she is taking will have no other source than the bottle or packet in which the drug has been prescribed. Unless the doctor has specifically requested otherwise all prescribed drugs should today be properly labelled with either the brand name or the generic name.

Any reader who wants to know more still about a product that has been prescribed for him will find it easy to obtain information by consulting one of the reference books listed on p. 341. Some or all of these books should be available in any local reference library.

Drugs included in the table

There are many thousands of drugs available, and I do not claim that this list is by any means comprehensive. It does, however, deal with many of the drugs used regularly by GPs and hospital doctors. I have omitted the very many drugs that are used in the treatment of rare diseases or that are only used in the operating theatre or research laboratory. I have compiled the list with the aid of many books, journals and private sources but one major basis for the collection is the second report of the World Health Organization Expert Committee, published as a booklet called *The selection of essential drugs* in the WHO Technical Report series. Drugs included in my list that also appear on the list compiled by these international experts are marked with a dagger symbol in the first column.

In the table branded drugs appear with an initial capital letter; generic drugs with an initial small letter, e.g. **Panadol** is branded; **paracetamol** is generic. Where brand name drugs are listed I have provided basic information about some of the pharmacological ingredients. I have done this for two reasons. First, many patients are confused by the fact that the drugs they are given sometimes seem to change. For example, patients used to taking Valium tablets may find themselves being given a prescription for diazepam tablets. With the aid of the drugs table the reader can see that diazepam is merely the generic name for the substance in Valium tablets. Similarly, a patient who thought he ought to be taking Penbritin capsules can see that there is no reason to worry if he is given a prescription for ampicillin. Second, inquisitive patients who want to know something more about the drug they are taking will find their investigations easier if the constituents of the product have been identified. For example, the patient given a prescription for Veganin can see that Veganin contains aspirin, paracetamol and codeine phosphate.

Every attempt has been made to ensure that all the information in this section is accurate. However, it is inevitably incomplete. I have listed the main ingredients of branded products, but formulations may change from time to time and for practical reasons the composition of liquid medicines, skin preparations and so on may be different from the composition of the same drug when it is available as tablets or capsules.

In addition to providing basic information about the composition of branded drugs I have included the name of the manufacturer concerned (in brackets after the name of the drug). I see no reason why patients should not communicate directly with manufacturers if they require specific advice about drugs. (Addresses of drug companies appear on pp. 285–94.)

Forms in which drugs are prescribed

The term 'medicine' is used in the table to describe a drug that is sold and dispensed in liquid form suitable for oral use, as opposed to being available as tablets, capsules, injection, drops, aerosol spray, suppositories, mouth-wash or skin preparation. The term 'skin preparation' is used to cover creams, ointments, lotions, pastes, and so on (see 'Glossary of pharma-ceutical terms'. I have tried to make the list of 'forms' as complete as possible but companies are always producing variations on existing themes.

Uses

The use to which specific drugs are put vary from doctor to doctor and from patient to patient but I have attempted to give a very brief (and sometimes inevitably generalized) guide to the types of disorder treated with specific named products, or indicated the effect (e.g. laxative, analgesic, antacid, anti-inflammatory etc.; see 'Glossary of Pharmaceutical terms', pp. 280ff.) that the product is intended to have. I must stress that,

223

because a product is described as having one specific purpose, it does not necessarily mean that the drug will not, under certain circumstances, be used for other purposes.

Side effects

Some guides to prescription drugs conscientiously list all the side effects most commonly associated with specific products, but in general I have not done so here. The side effects that I have listed and associated with specific drugs (in the third column of the table) are particularly notable ones that have been reported; there may be many others that have never been reported. The truth is, I'm afraid, that any patient taking any drug might develop any side effect. Some side effects may be more common, but that does not mean that others are unknown or impossible, and it would be dangerous to suggest that certain drugs are associated only with certain side effects (see 'Unwanted effects of drugs', p. 210).

Coded drugs

Finally, in the third column of the table, I have indicated which drugs are coded (controlled under the Misuse of Drugs Act).

† indicates a drug appearing on the list compiled by the World Health Organization Expert Committee

acetazolamide†	tablets	used in the treatment of glaucoma, fluid retention
acetylsalicylic acid† *see* aspirin		
Actal (Winthrop) sodium polyhydroxyaluminium monocarbonate hexitol complex	tablets, medicine	an antacid
Actidil (Wellcome) triprolidine	tablets, medicine	used in the treatment of allergy problems; may cause drowsiness
Actifed (Wellcome) triprolidine, pseudoephedrine. Actifed compound linctus also contains codeine phosphate	tablets, medicine	used in the treatment of respiratory and nasal congestion; may cause drowsiness
Acupan (Carnegie Medical) nefopam hydrochloride	tablets, injection	an analgesic
Adcortyl (Squibb) triamcinolone acetonide (a steroid)	skin preparation	an anti-inflammatory; used in the treatment of skin conditions like dermatitis
adrenaline (a hormone)	injection, aerosol	used in the treatment of bronchospasm (e.g. in asthma) and acute anaphylactic shock reactions
Agarol (Warner) liquid paraffin, phenolphthalein, agar	medicine	a laxative
Aldactone (Searle) spironolactone	tablets	a diuretic
Aldomet (MSD) methyldopa	tablets, injection	used in the treatment of high blood pressure
Algipan (Wyeth) methyl nicotinate, histamine dihydrochloride, glycol salicylate, capsicum oleoresin	skin preparation	used in the treatment of rheumatism

---

With some drugs some side effects are common. But remember that all drugs may have any number of possible side effects; see p. 210

Allbee with C (Robins) thiamine, riboflavine, pyridoxine, nicotinamide, calcium pantothenate, ascorbic acid	capsules, medicine	used in the treatment of vitamin deficiencies and as a general tonic
allopurinol†	tablets	used in the treatment of gout
Aludrox (Wyeth) aluminium hydroxide	tablets, medicine	an antacid
aluminium hydroxide†	tablets, medicine	an antacid
Alupent (Boehringer Ingelheim) orciprenaline	tablets, medicine, aerosol, injection	used in the treatment of bronchospasm (e.g. in asthma and bronchitis)
amantadine	capsules, medicine	used in the treatment of Parkinson's disease; it is said to have anti-viral properties making it useful in the prevention of 'flu
Amesec (Lilly) aminophylline, ephedrine	capsules	used in the treatment of asthma
Amfipen (Brocades) ampicillin	capsules, medicine	an anti-infective
amiloride†	tablets	a diuretic
aminophylline†	tablets, suppositories, injection	used in the treatment of asthma and heart failure
amitryptyline†	tablets, capsules, injection	used in the treatment of depression, anxiety and bed wetting in children; causes dry mouth, sleepiness etc.
Amoxil (Bencard) amoxycillin	tablets, capsules, medicine, injection	an anti-infective
ampicillin†	capsules, medicine, injection	an anti-infective
Amytal (Lilly) amylobarbitone (a barbiturate)	tablets	a sedative and hypnotic
Anacal (Luitpold-Werk) heparinoid, prednisolone, lauromacrogol, hexachlorophane	suppositories, skin preparation	used in the treatment of piles etc.

Andursil (Geigy) aluminium hydroxide, magnesium carbonate, dimethicone	tablets, medicine	an antacid
Anovlar 21 (Schering) oral contraceptive *see* p. 269		
Antepar (Wellcome) piperazine	tablets, medicine	used in the treatment of worms
Anthisan (May & Baker) mepyramine	tablets, medicine, skin preparation	used in the treatment of allergy problems; can cause drowsiness if taken orally
Antoin (Cox) aspirin, codeine phosphate, caffeine	tablets	a pain reliever
Anturan (Geigy) sulphinpyrazone	tablets	used in the treatment of gout
Anusol HC (Warner) hydrocortisone (a steroid), benzyl benzoate, bismuth, resorcinol, Peru balsam, zinc oxide	skin preparation, suppositories	used in the treatment of hemorrhoids
Anxon (Beecham) ketazolam (a benzodiazepine)	capsules	used in the treatment of anxiety
Apisate (Wyeth) diethylpropion, thiamine, riboflavine, pyridoxine, nicotinamide	tablets	used in the treatment of obesity
Apresoline (CIBA) hydralazine hydrochloride	tablets, injection	used in the treatment of high blood pressure
Aprinox (Boots) bendrofluazide	tablets	a diuretic
ascorbic acid† (vitamin C)	tablets	used in the treatment of scurvy; no other proven use
Asilone (Berk) aluminium hydroxide, dimethicone	tablets, medicine	an antacid

---

**With some drugs some side effects are common. But remember that all
drugs may have any number of possible side effects; see p. 210**

aspirin†	tablets, gum	used in the treatment of mild to moderate pain and in the treatment of arthritis as a long-term anti-inflammatory
Atensine (Berk) diazepam (a benzodiazepine)	tablets	used in the treatment of anxiety
Ativan (Wyeth) lorazepam (a benzodiazepine)	tablets, injection	used in the treatment of anxiety
Atromid S (ICI) clofibrate	capsules	sometimes used to lower level of cholesterol in blood
atropine†	tablets, drops, injection	an anticholinergic; effects vary
Augmentin (Beecham) potassium clavulanate, amoxycillin	tablets	an anti-infective
Bactrim (Roche) trimethoprim, sulphamethoxazole	capsules, medicine, injection	an anti-infective
Baratol (Wyeth) indoramin	tablets	used in the treatment of high blood pressure
barbiturates	tablets, capsules	group of drugs formerly used as sedatives, hypnotics and tranquillizers, and now largely replaced by the benzodiazepines which are thought by some doctors to be safer; still widely used in treatment of epilepsy
Baycaron (Bayer) mefruside	tablets	a diuretic
Bayolin (Bayer) heparinoid, glycol salicylate, benzyl nicotinate	embrocation	used in the treatment of rheumatic conditions
BC 500 (Ayerst) thiamine, riboflavine, nicotinamide, pyridoxine, calcium pantothenate cyanocobalamin, ascorbic acid	tablets	used in the prevention and treatment of vitamin deficiency
BCG vaccine†	injection	used to provide protection against tuberculosis

228

beclomethasone† (a steroid)	skin preparation, aerosol	as a skin preparation used to control inflammatory and allergic problems, and as an inhalant used in the treatment of asthma
Becotide (A & H) beclomethasone (a steroid)	aerosol	used in the treatment of asthma
Benadryl (Parke Davis) diphenhydramine	capsules	used in the treatment of allergy problems; can cause drowsiness
Benemid (MSD) probenecid	tablets	used in the treatment of gout
Benoral (Winthrop) benorylate	tablets, medicine	a pain reliever
Benoxyl 5 and **10** (Stiefel) benzoyl peroxide	skin preparation	used in the treatment and prevention of acne
Benylin Expectorant (Parke Davis) diphenhydramine, ammonium chloride, sodium citrate, menthol	medicine	used in the treatment of coughs; can cause drowsiness
benzodiazepines	tablets, medicine, injection	group of drugs with wide range of effects on central nervous system used as sedatives, tranquillizers, anaesthetic agents, muscle relaxants, hypnotics etc.; can produce various side effects including drowsiness
benzoic acid†	application	an anti-infective
benzyl benzoate†	application	an anti-infective; used in the treatment of scabies
benzylpenicillin†	tablets, medicine, injection	an anti-infective
Berkolol (Berk) propranolol	tablets	used in the treatment of heart conditions such as irregular heartbeat and angina

With some drugs some side effects are common. But remember that all drugs may have any number of possible side effects; see p. 210

Beta-cardone (Duncan, Flockhart) sotalol	tablets, injection	used in the treatment of heart conditions such as irregular heartbeat and angina
Betadine (Napp) povidone iodine	skin preparation	an anti-infective
Betaloc (Astra) metoprolol	tablets, injection	used in the treatment of heart conditions such as irregular heartbeat and angina
betamethasone† (a steroid)	tablets, skin preparation	*see* corticosteroids
Betim (Burgess) timolol	tablets	used in the treatment of angina and high blood pressure
Betnelan (Glaxo) betamethasone (a steroid)	tablets	*see* corticosteroids
Betnesol (Glaxo) betamethasone (a steroid)	tablets, injection, drops, skin preparation	*see* corticosteroids
Betnovate (Glaxo) betamethasone valerate (a steroid)	skin preparation	used in the treatment of a number of inflammatory conditions such as eczema
Biogastrone (Winthrop) carbenoxolone	tablets	used in the treatment of gastric ulcers
Bisolvon (Boehringer Ingelheim) bromhexine	tablets, medicine, injection	used in the treatment of conditions where sputum is troublesome
Blocadren (MSD) timolol	tablets	used in the treatment of angina and high blood pressure
Bolvidon (Organon) mianserin hydrochloride	tablets	used in the treatment of depression
Bradilan (Napp) nicofuranose	tablets	used in the treatment of bad circulation
Brasivol (Stiefel) aluminium oxide	skin preparation	used in the treatment and prevention of acne
Brevinor (Syntex) oral contraceptive *see* p. 269		

Bricanyl (Astra) terbutaline	tablets, medicine, aerosol, injection	used in the treatment of congestion and bronchospasm (e.g. in asthma)
Bronchodil (Keymer) reproterol	tablets, aerosol	used in the treatment of asthma etc.
Brovon (Napp) adrenaline, atropine, papaverine	inhalant	used in the treatment of bronchospasm (e.g. in asthma)
Broxil (Beecham) phenethicillin	tablets, capsules, medicine	an anti-infective
Brufen (Boots) ibuprofen	tablets, medicine	used in the treatment of rheumatism and arthritis
Burinex (Leo) bumetanide	tablets, injection	a diuretic
Butacote (Geigy) phenylbutazone	tablets	used in the treatment of inflammatory diseases such as arthritis
Butazolidin (Geigy) phenylbutazone	suppositories, injection, tablets	used in the treatment of inflammatory diseases such as arthritis
Caladryl (Parke Davis) calamine, camphor, diphenhydramine	skin preparation	used to relieve irritated or inflamed skin
calamine	skin preparation	used to relieve irritated or inflamed skin
calcium carbonate†	tablets, powder	an antacid
Calmurid (Pharmacia) urea	skin preparation	used in the treatment of dry skin and eczema
Calpol (Calmic) paracetamol	medicine	a pain reliever
Canesten (Bayer) clotrimazole	tablets, skin preparation	an anti-infective
Capitol (Dermal) benzalkonium chloride	skin preparation	used in the treatment of dandruff and other scalp disorders

---

**With some drugs some side effects are common. But remember that all
drugs may have any number of possible side effects; see p. 210**

carbamazepine†	tablets, medicine	used as an anti-convulsant in the treatment of epilepsy and in the treatment of trigeminal neuralgia (type of face pain); can cause dizziness, drowsiness, rash
Catapres (Boehringer Ingelheim) clonidine	tablets, capsules, injection	used in the treatment of high blood pressure
Caved S (Tillotts) deglycyrrhizinized liquorice, aluminium hydroxide, magnesium carbonate, sodium bicarbonate	tablets	used in the treatment of peptic ulcers etc.
Ceanel (Quinoderm) phenylethyl alcohol, cetrimide, undecenoic acid, hydrous wool fat	skin preparation	used in the treatment of dermatitis of the scalp
Celevac (WBP) methylcellulose	tablets, granules	a laxative and anti-obesity drug
Ceporex (Glaxo) cephalexin	capsules, tablets, medicine	an anti-infective
Ceporin (Glaxo) cephaloridine	injection	an anti-infective
Cerumol (LAB) paradichlorobenzene, chlorbutol, turpentine	drops	used to remove ear wax
Cetavlon (ICI) cetrimide	skin preparation	used in the treatment of dandruff
Cetiprin (KabiVitrum) emepronium bromide	tablets	used for bladder control
charcoal†	powder, granules	used as an absorbent for poisons
Chendol (Weddel) chenodeoxycholic acid	capsules	used like chenodeoxycholic acid
chenodeoxycholic acid	capsules	sometimes used in treatment of gall stone disease since it dissolves some types of gall stones, obviating need for surgery
chloramphenicol†	capsules, medicine, injection, powder, drops	an anti-infective; most commonly used as eye drops in the treatment of conjunctivitis

chlordiazepoxide (a benzodiazepine)	tablets, capsules, injection	used in the treatment of anxiety, depression etc.
chlorhexidine†	skin preparation, mouthwash	an anti-infective
chlormethiazole	tablets, capsules, mixture	a hypnotic and sedative
Chloromycetin (Parke Davis) chloramphenicol	drops, ointment	an anti-infective
chloroquine†	tablets, medicine, injection	most commonly used in the prevention and treatment of malaria
chlorpheniramine†	tablets, medicine, injection	an anti-histamine; used in the treatment of allergies; commonly causes drowsiness
chlorpromazine†	tablets, medicine, injection, suppositories	a powerful tranquillizer; used in the treatment of severe mental disorders
chlorpropamide	tablets	used in the treatment of diabetes
chlorthalidone†	tablets	a diuretic
Choledyl (Warner) choline theophyllinate	tablets, medicine	used in the treatment of bronchospasm (e.g. in asthma)
cimetidine	tablets, medicine, injection	used in the treatment of peptic ulcers
Claradin (Nicholas) aspirin	tablets	a pain reliever
clomiphene†	tablets	used in the treatment of infertility; may increase the chances of multiple birth
cloxacillin†	capsules, medicine, injection	an anti-infective

**With some drugs some side effects are common. But remember that all
drugs may have any number of possible side effects; see p. 210**

coal tar†	application	used in the treatment of psoriasis and eczema
codeine†	tablets, medicine, injection	used as a pain killer, a cough suppressant and an anti-diarrhoeal
Codis (Reckitt & Colman) aspirin, codeine phosphate	tablets	a pain reliever
colchicine†	tablets	used in the treatment of acute gout
Colofac (Duphar) mebeverine hydrochloride	tablets	used in the treatment of gastro-intestinal spasm
Conova (Searle) oral contraceptive see p. 269		
Corgard (Squibb) nadolol	tablets	a beta blocker; used in the treatment of angina and high blood pressure
Corlan (Glaxo) hydrocortisone (a steroid)	tablets	used in the treatment of mouth ulcers
Cortelan (Glaxo) cortisone (a steroid)	tablets	*see* corticosteroids
corticosteroids (abbr. steroids)	tablets, injection, drops, skin preparation, aerosol	a group of powerful anti-inflammatory drugs; used in replacement therapy and the suppression of disease processes; used in the treatment of arthritis, asthma, skin diseases such as eczema; they can be dangerous, so should always be taken under strict supervision and should not be stopped suddenly; dosage should be adjusted if any other disease process becomes apparent; steroids can cause stomach upsets such as indigestion
Cortistab (Boots) cortisone (a steroid)	tablets, injection	*see* corticosteroids
co-trimoxazole	tablets, medicine, injection	an anti-infective
Crystapen V (Glaxo) penicillin V	tablets, medicine	an anti-infective

cyanocobalamin (vitamin B12)	injection	used in the treatment of vitamin B12 deficiency
Cyclo-progynova (Schering) hormones	tablets	used in the treatment of menopausal symptoms
Cyclospasmol (Brocades) cyclandelate	tablets, capsules, medicine	used in the treatment of poor circulation
Cytamen (Glaxo) cyanocobalamin	injection	used in the treatment of vitamin B12 deficiency
Dalacin C (Upjohn) clindamycin	capsules, medicine, injection	an anti-infective
Dalmane (Roche) flurazepam (a benzodiazepine)	capsules	a hypnotic
Daraprim (Wellcome) pyrimethamine	tablets	an anti-malarial
Debendox (Merrell) dicyclomine hydrochloride, doxylamine succinate, pyridoxine hydrochloride	tablets	used to prevent nausea and vomiting
debrisoquine	tablets	used in the treatment of high blood pressure
Decaserpyl (Roussel) methoserpidine	tablets	used in the treatment of high blood pressure
Declinax (Roche) debrisoquine	tablets	used in the treatment of high blood pressure
Demulen 50 (Searle) oral contraceptive *see* p. 269		
De-Nol (Brocades) tri-potassium di-citrato bismuthate	medicine	used in the treatment of peptic ulcers
Depo-medrone (Upjohn) methylprednisolone (a steroid)	injection	*see* corticosteroids
Depronal SA (Warner) dextropropoxyphene	capsules	a pain reliever
Dequadin (Farley) dequalinium	lozenges	used in the treatment of infections of the mouth and throat

---

With some drugs some side effects are common. But remember that all drugs may have any number of possible side effects; see p. 210

Dermovate (Glaxo)
clobetasol propionate
(a powerful steroid)

skin
preparation

used in the treatment of
skin problems such as
psoriasis and eczema which
do not respond to less
powerful steroids

Deteclo (Lederle)
chlortetracycline,
tetracycline,
demeclocycline

tablets,
medicine

an anti-infective

Dettol (Reckitt & Colman)
chloroxylenol

skin
preparation

an anti-infective

dexamethasone†
(a steroid)

tablets,
injection

see corticosteroids

Dexedrine (Smith, Kline
& French)
dexamphetamine

tablets

a stimulant; coded drug

dextropropoxyphene

capsules

a pain reliever

DF118 (Duncan, Flockhart)
dihydrocodeine tartrate

tablets,
medicine,
injection

a pain reliever;
injection is coded drug

Diabinese (Pfizer)
chlorpropamide

tablets

used in the treatment of
diabetes

Diamox (Lederle)
acetazolamide

tablets,
injection

a diuretic

diazepam ‖
(a benzodiazepine)

tablets,
medicine,
injection

a tranquillizer; widely used
in the treatment of mild
anxiety states and also in
the treatment of epilepsy
and as an anaesthetic

Dibotin (Winthrop)
phenformin

tablets,
capsules

used in the treatment of
diabetes

Diconal (Calmic)
dipipanone

tablets

a pain reliever; coded drug

Difflam (Carnegie Medical)
benzydamine

skin
preparation

used in the treatment of
musculo-skeletal pain and
inflammation

digoxin†

tablets,
medicine,
injection

used in the control of heart
failure

Dimotane Expectorant
(Robins)
brompheniramine,
guaiphenesin, phenylephrine,
phenylpropanolamine

medicine

used in the treatment of
coughs; can cause
drowsiness

Dimotane LA (Robins) brompheniramine	tablets, medicine	used in the treatment of allergy problems; can cause drowsiness
Dimotapp LA (Robins) brompheniramine, phenylephrine, phenylpropanolamine	tablets, medicine	used in the treatment of catarrh, rhinitis and sinusitis; can cause drowsiness
Dioralyte (Armour) sodium chloride, potassium chloride, sodium bicarbonate, dextrose monohydrate	sachets	given by mouth to correct the fluid and electrolyte loss in children and adults that may occur with diarrhoea
diphtheria antitoxin†	injection	used to provide protection against diphtheria
diphtheria-pertussis-tetanus vaccine†	injection	used to provide protection against diphtheria, whooping cough (pertussis) and tetanus
diphtheria-tetanus vaccine†	injection	used to provide protection against diphtheria and tetanus
Distalgesic (Dista) mixture of dextropropoxyphene and paracetamol	tablets	a pain reliever
Diurexan (Merck) xipamide	tablets	a diuretic; used in the treatment of high blood pressure and whenever a diuretic is needed
Dixarit (WBP) clonidine	tablets	used in the treatment of migraine and menopausal flushing
Dolasan (Lilly) dextropropoxyphene, aspirin	tablets	a pain reliever
Dolobid (Morson) diflunisal	tablets	a pain reliever
Doloxene (Lilly) dextropropoxyphene	capsules	a pain reliever
Dorbanex (Riker) danthron	capsules, medicine	a laxative
Doriden (CIBA) glutethimide	tablets	a hypnotic

With some drugs some side effects are common. But remember that all drugs may have any number of possible side effects; see p. 210

dothiepin	tablets, capsules	used in the treatment of depression
doxycycline† (a member of the tetracycline family)	capsules, medicine	an anti-infective
Drapolene (Wellcome) benzalkonium chloride, cetrimide	skin preparation	an anti-infective; used to prevent ammonia dermatitis caused by urine
Dulcodos (Boehringer Ingelheim) bisacodyl, docusate sodium	tablets	a laxative
Dulcolax (Boehringer Ingelheim) bisacodyl	tablets, suppositories	a laxative
Duo-Autohaler (Riker) isoprenaline, phenylephrine	aerosol	used in the treatment of bronchospasm (e.g. in asthma)
Duogastrone (Winthrop) carbenoxolone	capsules	used in the treatment of duodenal ulcer
Duphalac (Duphar) lactulose	medicine	a laxative
Duphaston (Duphar) dydrogesterone (progesterone hormone)	tablets	used in the treatment of premenstrual syndrome, painful periods, threatened abortion and endometriosis
Duromine (Carnegie Medical) phentermine	capsules	used in the treatment of obesity
Durophet (Riker) amphetamine, dexamphetamine	capsules	used as a stimulant and anti-obesity drug; coded drug
Duvadilan (Duphar) isoxsuprine	tablets, capsules, injection	used in the treatment of poor circulation
Dyazide (Smith, Kline & French) triamterene, hydrochlorothiazide	tablets	a diuretic
Eczederm (Quinoderm) calamine	skin preparation	used to relieve irritated or inflamed skin
Efcortelan (Glaxo) hydrocortisone (a steroid)	skin preparation	used in the treatment of many skin conditions including eczema

Effico (Pharmax) thiamine, nicotinamide, caffeine, gentian infusion	medicine	a tonic
Epanutin (Parke Davis) phenytoin	tablets, capsules, medicine, injection	used in the treatment of epilepsy
ephedrine hydrochloride†	tablets, medicine	used in the treatment of wheeziness and nasal congestion
Epilim (Labaz) sodium valproate	tablets, medicine	used in the treatment of epilepsy
epinephrine† *see* adrenaline		
Equagesic (Wyeth) ethoheptazine, meprobamate, aspirin	tablets	a pain reliever
Equanil (Wyeth) meprobamate	tablets	used in the treatment of anxiety
ergocalciferol† (vitamin D)	tablets, capsules, medicine	used only in the treatment of vitamin D deficiency (e.g. rickets)
ergometrine†	tablets, injection	has effects on the womb; used to control bleeding after birth or abortion
ergotamine†	tablets, aerosol, suppositories	used in the treatment of migraine; careful control needed because of risks of gangrene with too much use
Erythrocin (Abbott) erythromycin	tablets, medicine, injection	an anti-infective
erythromycin†	tablets, medicine, injection	an anti-infective
Erythroped (Abbott) erythromycin	medicine	an anti-infective
Esoderm (Napp) gamma benzene hexachloride	skin preparation	used in the treatment of head and body lice and scabies

---

With some drugs some side effects are common. But remember that all
drugs may have any number of possible side effects; see p. 210

ethambutol hydrochloride†	tablets	used in the treatment of tuberculosis
ethinyloestradiol† (an oestrogen hormone)	tablets	used in the treatment of menopausal symptoms and as an oral contraceptive (*see* p. 269)
ethosuximide†	capsules, medicine	used in the treatment of minor seizures
Euglucon (Roussel) glibenclamide	tablets	used in the treatment of diabetes
Eugynon 30 (Schering) **Eugynon 50** (Schering) oral contraceptives *see* p. 269		
Euhypnos (Farmitalia) temazepam (a benzodiazepine)	capsules	a hypnotic
Eumovate (Glaxo) clobetasone butyrate (a steroid)	drops, skin preparation	used in the treatment of skin conditions including eczema and inflammatory eye conditions
Expansyl (Smith, Kline & French) ephedrine, diphenylpyraline, trifluoperazine	capsules	used in the prevention and treatment of bronchospasm (e.g. in asthma)
Fabahistin (Bayer) mebhydrolin	tablets, medicine	used in the treatment of allergy problems; can cause drowsiness
Fefol (Smith, Kline & French ferrous sulphate, folic acid	capsules	used in the treatment and prevention of iron and folic acid deficiency
Feldene (Pfizer) piroxicam	capsules	used in the treatment of inflammatory diseases such as arthritis
Femulen (Searle) oral contraceptive *see* p. 269		
Fenopron (Dista) fenoprofen	tablets	a pain reliever
Fenostil Retard (Zyma) dimethindene maleate	tablets	an anti-histamine; used in the treatment of allergy problems; may cause drowsiness
Fentazin (Allen and Hanburys) perphenazine	tablets, injection	used in the treatment of anxiety etc.

240

Feospan (Smith, Kline & French) ferrous sulphate	capsules	used in the treatment and prevention of iron deficiency anaemia
Ferrograd C (Abbott) ferrous sulphate, ascorbic acid	tablets	used in the treatment and prevention of iron deficiency anaemia
Ferro-Gradumet (Abbott) ferrous sulphate	tablets	used in the treatment and prevention of iron deficiency anaemia
ferrous salts† (include ferrous fumarate, ferrous gluconate, ferrous succinate, ferrous sulphate)	tablets, capsules, medicine	used in the treatment and prevention of iron deficiency anaemia
Fersamal (Glaxo) ferrous fumarate	tablets, medicine	used in the treatment and prevention of iron deficiency anaemia
Fesovit (Smith, Kline & French) ferrous sulphate, ascorbic acid, thiamine, riboflavine, pyridoxine, nicotinamide, calcium pantothenate	capsules	used in the treatment and prevention of iron deficiency anaemia when supplementary vitamins are also required
Filon (Berk) phenbutrazate, phenmetrazine	tablets	used in the treatment of obesity; coded drug
Flagyl (May & Baker) metronidazole	tablets, suppositories, injection	an anti-infective
Floxapen (Beecham) flucloxacillin	capsules, medicine, injection	an anti-infective
Fluanxol (Lundbeck) flupenthixol dihydrochloride	tablets	used in the treatment of depression etc.
fludrocortisone† (a steroid)	tablets	used in the treatment of adrenal gland malfunctions
fluphenazine†	injection	used in the treatment of schizophrenia and other serious mental disorders
folic acid†	tablets	used in the treatment and prevention of specific types of anaemia

---

With some drugs some side effects are common. But remember that all drugs may have any number of possible side effects; see p. 210

Fortagesic (Winthrop) pentazocine, paracetamol	tablets	a pain reliever
Fortral (Winthrop) pentazocine	tablets, capsules, injection, suppositories	a pain reliever
Franol (Winthrop) ephedrine, theophylline, phenobarbitone (a barbiturate)	tablets, medicine	used in the treatment of bronchitis and asthma
Froben (Boots) flurbiprofen	tablets	used in the treatment of inflammatory diseases such as arthritis
frusemide†	tablets, injection	a diuretic
Fucidin (Leo) sodium fusidate	tablets, capsules, medicine, injection, skin preparation	an anti-infective
Furadantin (Eaton) nitrofurantoin	tablets, medicine	an anti-infective
Fybogel (Reckitt & Colman) ispaghula husk, sodium bicarbonate, citric acid	granules	a laxative
gamma benzene hydrochloride†	application	used in the treatment of scabies
Garoin (May & Baker) phenytoin, phenobarbitone (a barbiturate)	tablets	used to control epilepsy
Gastrils (Jackson) aluminium hydroxide, magnesium carbonate	pastilles	an antacid
Gaviscon (Reckitt & Colman) magnesium trisilicate, aluminium hydroxide, sodium bicarbonate etc.	tablets, granules, medicine	an antacid
Gelusil (Warner) aluminium hydroxide, magnesium trisilicate	tablets, medicine	an antacid
gentamicin†	injection	an anti-infective

gentian and alkali mixture	medicine	a traditional tonic
Glucophage (Rona) metformin	tablets	used in the treatment of diabetes
glyceryl trinitrate†	tablets	used in the treatment and prevention of angina; tablets are dissolved under the tongue; can cause headaches
griseofulvin†	tablets, medicine	an anti-infective
Gyno-Daktarin (Janssen) miconazole nitrate	skin preparation, suppositories	an anti-infective
Gynovlar 21 (Schering) oral contraceptive *see* p. 269		
Halcion (Upjohn) triazolam (a benzodiazepine)	tablets	a hypnotic
haloperidol†	tablets, medicine, injection	a major tranquillizer; used in the treatment of severe mental disorders
Harmogen (Abbott) piperazine oestrone (an oestrogen hormone)	tablets	used in the treatment of menopause symptoms
Haymine (Pharmax) chlorpheniramine, ephedrine	tablets	used in the treatment of allergy problems; can cause drowsiness
Heminevrin (Astra) chlormethiazole edisylate	capsules, medicine	a sedative
heparin†	injection	used in the treatment and prevention of blood-clotting
Hexopal (Winthrop) inositol nicotinate	tablets, medicine	used in the treatment of poor circulation
Hibitane (ICI) chlorhexidine	skin preparation	an anti-infective
Histryl (Smith, Kline & French) diphenylpyraline	capsules	used in the treatment of allergy problems; can cause drowsiness
hormones *see* p. 268		

With some drugs some side effects are common. But remember that all drugs may have any number of possible side effects; see p. 210

hydralazine†	tablets, injection	dilates the blood vessels so used in the treatment of high blood pressure; can cause dizziness
hydrochlorthiazide†	tablets	a diuretic; sometimes also used in the treatment of high blood pressure
hydrocortisone† (a steroid)	tablets, injection	*see* corticosteroids
hydroxocobalamin† (vitamin B12)	injection	used in the treatment of vitamin B12 deficiency, which is caused by inability to absorb vitamin orally, so it is given by injection
Hygroton (Geigy) chlorthalidone	tablets	a diuretic
Hypon (Calmic) aspirin, codeine phosphate, caffeine	tablets	a pain reliever
Hypovase (Pfizer) prazosin	tablets	used in the treatment of heart failure and high blood pressure
ibuprofen†	tablets, medicine	used as a pain reliever and in the treatment of inflammation associated with rheumatic and like diseases
Icipen (ICI) penicillin V	tablets, medicine	an anti-infective
Ilosone (Dista) erythromycin	tablets, capsules, medicine	an anti-infective
imipramine	tablets, medicine, injection	used in the treatment of depression and bed-wetting
Imodium (Janssen) loperamide	capsules, medicine	used in the treatment of diarrhoea
Imperacin (ICI) oxytetracycline	tablets, medicine	an anti-infective
Inderal (ICI) propranolol hydrochloride	tablets, capsules, injection	used in the treatment of high blood pressure, anxiety and thyrotoxicosis; must not be stopped suddenly

Indocid (Morson) indomethacin	capsules, medicine, suppositories	used in the treatment of inflammatory diseases such as arthritis
indomethacin†	capsules, medicine, suppositories	used in the treatment of inflammatory diseases such as arthritis
influenza vaccine†	injection	used to provide protection against influenza
insulin† (various kinds available)	injection	used in the treatment of diabetes mellitus (sugar diabetes)
Intal (Fisons) sodium cromoglycate	capsules for inhalation	used in the prevention of asthma
Integrin (Sterling) oxypertine	tablets, capsules	used in the treatment of anxiety etc.
interferon	injection	a controversial, expensive drug said to have anti- cancer effect in some circumstances
iodine†	skin preparation	used as a skin disinfectant
ipecacuanha†	medicine	used to induce vomiting after poisoning and also in cough mixtures
Ipral (Squibb) trimethoprim	tablets, medicine	an anti-infective
Irofol C (Abbott) ferrous sulphate, folic acid, ascorbic acid	tablets	used in the treatment and prevention of iron deficiency anaemia in pregnancy
Iso-Autohaler (Riker) isoprenaline	aerosol	used in the treatment of bronchospasm (e.g. in asthma)
Isogel (A & H) ispaghula husk	granules	a laxative
Isoket Retard (Sanol) isosorbide dinitrate	tablets	used in the prevention of angina
isoniazid†	tablets, medicine injection	used in the treatment of tuberculosis

---

**With some drugs some side effects are common. But remember that all
drugs may have any number of possible side effects; see p. 210**

isoprenaline hydrochloride†	tablets, injection	used in the treatment of slow heartbeat
isoprenaline sulphate	tablets, spray, aerosol	used in the treatment of bronchospasm
Isordil Tembids (Ayerst) isosorbide dinitrate	capsules	used in the prevention and treatment of angina
isosorbide dinitrate†	tablets, capsules	used in the prevention and treatment of angina; tablets may be dissolved under the tongue
Ivax (Boots) neomycin, kaolin	medicine	used in the treatment of diarrhoea
kaolin mixture	medicine	used in the treatment of diarrhoea; sometimes prescribed in mixture with morphine
Keflex (Lilly) cephalexin	tablets, capsules, medicine	an anti-infective
Kelfizine (Farmitalia) sulfametopyrazine	tablets, medicine	an anti-infective
Lacticare (Stiefel) lactic acid, sodium pyrrolidone carboxylate	skin preparation	used in the treatment of dry skin
laetrile laevo mandelonitrile (found in the stones of apricots, peaches, plums)	injection	said to kill cancer cells; very controversial and not available on prescription
Lanoxin (Wellcome) digoxin	tablets, medicine, injection	used in the treatment of heart failure
Largactil (May & Baker) chlorpromazine hydrochloride	tablets, medicine, injection	used in the treatment of many mental disorders
Lasix (Hoechst) frusemide	tablets, medicine, injection	a diuretic
Lederfen (Lederle) fenbufen	capsules	used in the treatment of inflammatory diseases such as arthritis
Ledermycin (Lederle) demeclocycline	tablets, capsules, medicine	an anti-infective

Lenium (Winthrop) selenium sulphide	skin preparation	used in the treatment of dandruff
Lentizol (Warner) amitriptyline hydrochloride	capsules	used in the treatment of depression
Leo K (Leo) potassium chloride	tablets	used in the prevention and treatment of potassium depletion; often prescribed in conjunction with diuretic therapy since some diuretics produce an excessive loss of potassium from the body
Levius (Farmitalia) aspirin	tablets	a pain reliever
levodopa†	tablets, capsules	used in the treatment of Parkinson's disease
Librium (Roche) chlordiazepoxide (a benzodiazepine)	tablets, capsules, injection	used in the treatment of anxiety, depression etc.
Limbitrol (Roche) chlordiazepoxide (a benzodiazepine), amitriptyline	capsules	used in the treatment of anxiety, depression etc.
Linctifed (Wellcome) triprolidine, pseudoephedrine, codeine phosphate, guaiphenesin	medicine	used in the treatment of coughs and congestion; can cause drowsiness
Lioresal (CIBA) baclofen	tablets	used in the treatment of muscle spasticity
lithium carbonate†	tablets	used as a mood-regulating drug to control depression and mania
Lobak (Winthrop) chlormezanone, paracetamol	tablets	a pain reliever
Locoid (Brocades) hydrocortisone 17 butyrate (a steroid)	skin preparation	used in the treatment of inflammatory skin conditions
Loestrin 20 (Parke Davis) **Logynon** (Schering) oral contraceptives *see* p. 269		
Lomotil (Searle) diphenoxylate, atropine sulphate	tablets, medicine	used in the treatment of diarrhoea

---

With some drugs some side effects are common. But remember that all drugs may have any number of possible side effects; see p. 210

Lopresor (Geigy) metoprolol	tablets	used in the treatment of heart conditions
lorazepam (a benzodiazepine)	tablets, injection	a tranquillizer
Lorexane (ICI) gamma benzene hydrochloride	skin preparation	used in the treatment of scabies and lice
Lotussin (Searle) diphenhydramine, dextromethorphan, ephedrine, guaiphenesin	medicine	used in the treatment of coughs; can cause drowsiness
Ludiomil (CIBA) maprotiline hydrochloride	tablets	used in the treatment of depression
Maalox (Radiol) aluminium hydroxide, magnesium hydroxide	tablets, medicine	an antacid
Magnapen (Beecham) ampicillin, flucloxacillin	capsules, medicine, injection	an anti-infective
magnesium hydroxide†	medicine	an antacid; can cause diarrhoea
mannitol†	injection	a powerful diuretic
Maxolon (Beecham) metoclopramide	tablets, medicine, injection	used in the treatment of stomach upsets of all kinds and to control nausea and vomiting
M & B 693 (May & Baker) sulphapyridine	tablets	an anti-infective
measles vaccine†	injection	used to provide protection against measles
mebendazole†	tablets, medicine	used in the treatment of parasitic worms
Medihaler Duo (Riker) isoprenaline, phenylephrine	aerosol	used in the treatment of bronchospasm (e.g. in asthma)
Medihaler Epi (Riker) adrenaline	aerosol	used in the treatment of bronchospasm (e.g. in asthma)
Medihaler Iso (Riker) isoprenaline	aerosol	used in the treatment of bronchospasm (e.g. in asthma)
Megaclor (Pharmax) clomocycline	capsules	an anti-infective

Melleril (Sandoz) thioridazine	tablets, medicine	used in the treatment of tension and a wide range of mental disorders
Menophase (Syntex) mestranol, norethisterone (hormones)	tablets	used in the treatment of menopausal symptoms
Meralen (Merrell) flufenamic acid	capsules	a pain reliever
Merbentyl (Merrell) dicyclomine hydrochloride	tablets, medicine	used in the treatment of intestinal spasm or colic
Metatone (Parke Davis) thiamine, glycerophosphates of calcium, manganese, potassium, sodium	medicine	a tonic
Methrazone (WBP) feprazone	capsules	used in the treatment of inflammatory diseases such as arthritis
methyldopa†	tablets, injection	used in the treatment of high blood pressure; may cause dry mouth, drowsiness, impotence
Metosyn (Stuart) fluocinonide (a steroid)	skin preparation	used in the treatment of inflammatory skin conditions
metronidazole†	tablets, suppositories	an anti-infective
mianserin	tablets	used in the treatment of depression
miconazole†	tablets, suppositories, skin preparation	an anti-infective
Microgynon 30 (Schering) **Micronor** (Ortho) **Microval** (Wyeth) oral contraceptives *see* p. 269		
Migraleve (International) buclizine dihydrochloride, paracetamol, codeine phosphate, docusate sodium	tablets	used in the treatment of migraine; can cause drowsiness

With some drugs some side effects are common. But remember that all
drugs may have any number of possible side effects; see p. 210

Migril (Wellcome) ergotamine, cyclizine, caffeine	tablets	used in the treatment of migraine
Minilyn (Organon) **Minovlar** (Schering) **Minovlar ED** (Schering) oral contraceptives *see* p. 269		
Mixogen (Organon) ethinyloestradiol, methyltestosterone (hormones)	tablets, injection	used in the treatment of menopausal symptoms
Modecate (Squibb) fluphenazine decanoate	injection	used in the treatment of mentally ill patients who are not reliable tablet-takers
Moditen (Squibb) fluphenazine hydrochloride	tablets	used in the treatment of anxiety etc.
Moducren (Morson) hydrochlorothiazide, amiloride hydrochloride, timolol maleate	tablets	used in the treatment of high blood pressure
Moduretic (MSD) amiloride, hydrochlorothiazide	tablets	a diuretic
Mogadon (Roche) nitrazepam (a benzodiazepine)	tablets, capsules	a hypnotic
Molipaxin (Roussel) trazadone hydrochloride	capsules	an anti-depressant
Monistat (Ortho) miconazole nitrate	skin preparation, suppositories	an anti-infective
Monotrim (Duphar) trimethoprim	tablets	an anti-infective used mostly for urinary tract and respiratory tract infections
morphine†	tablets, medicine, suppositories, injection	a powerful pain killer; addictive; coded drug
Motival (Squibb) nortriptyline, fluphenazine	tablets	used in the treatment of anxiety, depression etc.
MST-1 Continus (Napp) morphine sulphate	tablets	used in the treatment of severe pain; coded drug
Mucaine (Wyeth) oxethazaine, aluminium hydroxide, magnesium hydroxide	medicine	an antacid

Mucodyne (Berk) carbocisteine	capsules, medicine	used in the treatment of conditions involving excessive mucus
Multivite (Duncan, Flockhart) vitamin A, thiamine, ascorbic acid, calciferol	tablets	used in the treatment and prevention of vitamin deficiency
Myocrisin (May & Baker) sodium aurothiomalate	injections	used in the treatment of inflammatory diseases such as arthritis
Mysteclin (Squibb) tetracycline	tablets, capsules, medicine	an anti-infective
naloxone†	injection	used to treat morphine overdose
Naprosyn (Syntex) naproxen	tablets, medicine, suppositories	used in the treatment of inflammatory diseases such as arthritis
Navidrex (CIBA) cyclopenthiazide	tablets	a diuretic
Navidrex K (CIBA) cyclopenthiazide, potassium chloride	tablets	a diuretic; like many diuretics widely used in the treatment of high blood pressure
Negram (Sterling) nalidixic acid	tablets, medicine	an anti-infective
Nembutal (Abbott) pentobarbitone (a barbiturate)	capsules	a sedative and hypnotic
Neogest (Schering) oral contraceptive *see* p. 269		
Neo-Medrone (Upjohn) methylprednisolone, neomycin sulphate	skin preparation	used in the treatment of acne
neomycin†	tablets, medicine, drops, skin preparation	an anti-infective
Neo-naclex (Duncan, Flockhart) bendrofluazide	tablets	a diuretic

---

**With some drugs some side effects are common. But remember that all
drugs may have any number of possible side effects; see p. 210**

251

neostigmine†	tablets, injection	used in the diagnosis and treatment of myasthenia gravis
Nephril (Pfizer) polythiazide	tablets	a diuretic
Nicorette (Lundbeck) nicotine resin	chewing-gum	advocated as an aid for people trying to give up smoking
nicotinamide† (member of the vitamin B group)	tablets	*see* p. 278
nitrazepam (a benzodiazepine)	tablets, capsules	a hypnotic
nitrofurantoin†	tablets, capsules, medicine	an anti-infective; most commonly used in the treatment of urinary tract infections
Nobrium (Roche) medazepam (a benzodiazepine)	capsules	used in the treatment of anxiety etc.
Noctamid (Schering) lormetazepam (a benzodiazepine)	tablets	used in the treatment of insomnia
norethisterone† (progesterone hormone)	tablets	used in the treatment of bleeding, endometriosis and in the contraceptive pill
Norgeston (Schering) **Noriday** (Syntex) **Norimin** (Syntex) **Norinyl 1** (Syntex) **Norinyl 1/28** (Syntex) **Norlestrin** (Parke Davis) oral contraceptives *see* p. 269		
Normacol (Norgine) sterculia	granules	a laxative
Norval (Bencard) mianserin	tablets	used in the treatment of depression
Nuelin (Riker) theophylline	tablets, medicine	used in the treatment of bronchospasm (e.g. in asthma)
NuSeals Aspirin (Lilly) aspirin	tablets	a pain reliever

Nystan (Squibb) nystatin	tablets, medicine, skin preparation, suppositories	an anti-infective
nystatin†	tablets, medicine, suppositories, skin preparation	an anti-infective
Oilatum Cream (Stiefel) arachis oil	skin preparation	soothing substance for dry skin
Omnopon (Roche) papaveretum	tablets, injection	used as a pain reliever; coded drug
Opilon (Warner) thymoxamine	tablets, injection	used in the treatment of poor circulation
Opren (Dista) benoxaprofen	tablets	used in the treatment of inflammatory diseases such as arthritis
Optimine (Kirby-Warrick) azatadine	tablets, medicine	used in the treatment of allergy problems; may cause drowsiness
Orabase (Squibb) sodium carboxymethylcellulose, pectin, gelatin	skin preparation	used to protect and soothe the skin
Oraldene (Warner) hexetidine	mouthwash	an anti-infective; used in the treatment of mouth infections
Orbenin (Beecham) cloxacillin	capsules, medicine, injection	an anti-infective
Orlest 21 (Parke Davis) oral contraceptive *see* p. 269		
Orovite (Bencard) thiamine, riboflavine, pyridoxine, nicotinamide, ascorbic acid	tablets, medicine	used in the treatment of vitamin deficiencies
Ortho Novin 1/50 (Ortho) oral contraceptive *see* p. 269		

**With some drugs some side effects are common. But remember that all
drugs may have any number of possible side effects; see p. 210**

253

Orudis (May & Baker) ketoprofen	capsules, suppositories	used in the treatment of inflammatory diseases such as arthritis
Otosporin (Calmic) polymyxin, neomycin, hydrocortisone (a steroid)	drops	an anti-infective used in the treatment of ear infections
Otrivine (CIBA) xylometazoline	spray, drops	used in the treatment of nasal congestion
Otrivine Antistin (CIBA) xylometazoline, antazoline	drops, spray	used in the treatment of allergy problems
Ovran (Wyeth) **Ovran 30** (Wyeth) **Ovranette** (Wyeth) **Ovulen 50** (Searle) **Ovysmen** (Ortho) oral contraceptives *see* p. 269		
oxytocin† (a hormone)	injection	stimulates the womb muscles; used to induce labour
Pacitron (Berk) L-tryptophan	tablets	used in the treatment of depression
Palaprin (Nicholas) aloxiprin	tablets	used in the treatment of inflammatory diseases, such as arthritis, and as a pain reliever
Palfium (MCP) dextromoramide	tablets, suppositories, injection	a pain reliever; coded drug
Panadeine Co (Winthrop) paracetamol, codeine phosphate	tablets	a pain reliever
Panadol (Winthrop) paracetamol	tablets, medicine	a pain reliever
Panasorb (Winthrop) paracetamol	tablets	a pain reliever
paracetamol†	tablets, medicine	a pain reliever
Paracodol (Fisons) paracetamol, codeine phosphate	tablets	a pain reliever
Parahypon (Calmic) paracetamol, codeine phosphate, caffeine	tablets	a pain reliever

Paramol 118 (Duncan, Flockhart) paracetamol, dihydrocodeine tartrate	tablets	a pain reliever
Para-Seltzer (Wander) paracetamol, caffeine	tablets	a pain reliever
Paynocil (Beecham) aspirin, amino acetic acid	tablets	a pain reliever
Penbritin (Beecham) ampicillin	tablets, capsules, medicine, injection	an anti-infective
penicillamine†	tablets, capsules	used in the treatment of severe arthritis; nothing to do with penicillin
penicillin†	tablets, capsules, medicine, injection	an anti-infective
Penidural (Wyeth) benzathine penicillin	medicine, injection	an anti-infective
Penotrane (WBP) hydrargaphen	suppositories	an anti-infective
Periactin (MSD) cyproheptadine	tablets, medicine	used as an appetite stimulant and in the treatment of allergy problems; can cause drowsiness
Pernivit (Duncan, Flockhart) acetamenaphthone, nicotinic acid	tablets	used in the treatment of poor circulation and particularly chilblains
pethidine†	tablets, injection	used in the treatment of severe pain; coded drug
Phenergan (May & Baker) promethazine	tablets, medicine, injection, skin preparation	used in the treatment of allergy problems and in the treatment and prevention of nausea and vomiting; may cause drowsiness
phenobarbitone† (a barbiturate)	tablets, capsules, medicine	used in the treatment and prevention of epilepsy and also as a hypnotic

With some drugs some side effects are common. But remember that all drugs may have any number of possible side effects; see p. 210

Phensedyl (May & Baker) promethazine, codeine phosphate, ephedrine	medicine	used in the treatment of coughs; may cause drowsiness
phenylbutazone	tablets, suppositories, injections	used in the treatment of inflammatory diseases such as arthritis
phenytoin †	tablets, capsules, injection	used in the prevention and treatment of epilepsy
pHiso-Med (Winthrop) hexachlorophane	skin preparation	an anti-infective
Pholcomed (Medo) pholcodine, papaverine	medicine, pastilles	used in the treatment of coughs
Pholtex (Riker) pholcodine, phenyltoloxamine	medicine	used in the treatment of coughs; may cause drowsiness
Phyllocontin (Napp) aminophylline	tablets	used in the treatment of lung disorders, such as asthma, and heart disorders, such as heart failure
Physeptone (Wellcome) methadone	tablets, medicine, injection	a pain reliever; coded drug
pilocarpine †	drops	used in the treatment of eye conditions such as glaucoma
piperazine †	tablets, medicine	used in the treatment of worms
Piriton (A & H) chlorpheniramine	tablets, medicine, injection	used in the treatment of allergy problems; may cause drowsiness
poliomyelitis vaccine †	medicine, injection	used to provide protection against poliomyelitis
Polycrol (Nicholas) aluminium hydroxide, magnesium hydroxide, dimethicone	tablets, medicine	an antacid
Polytar (Stiefel) tar, coal tar, cade oil, arachis oil, oleyl alcohol	skin preparation	used in the treatment of skin conditions such as psoriasis
Ponderax (Servier) fenfluramine	capsules, tablets	used in the treatment of obesity
Ponstan (Parke Davis) mefenamic acid	capsules, medicine	a pain reliever

Posalfilin (Norgine)
salicylic acid, podophyllin | skin preparation | used in the treatment of warts

Praxilene (Lipha)
naftidrofuryl oxalate | capsules, injection | said to have value as blood vessel dilator; used in the treatment of conditions involving narrowing of the arteries (e.g. strokes, bad circulation)

Prednesol (Glaxo)
prednisolone (a steroid) | tablets | *see* corticosteroids

prednisolone†
(a steroid) | tablets, injection | *see* corticosteroids

prednisone
(a steroid) | tablets | *see* corticosteroids

Prefil (Norgine)
sterculia | granules | a laxative; used in the treatment of obesity

Pregaday (Glaxo)
ferrous fumarate, folic acid | tablets | used in the treatment and prevention of iron deficiency anaemia, specifically during pregnancy

Premarin (Ayerst)
conjugated oestrogen hormones | tablets | used in the treatment of menopausal symptoms

Premarin Vaginal Cream
(Ayerst) oestrogen hormones | skin preparation | used in the treatment of vaginitis etc.

Primalan (Smith & Nephew)
mequitazine | tablets | used in the treatment of allergy problems; may cause drowsiness

Primolut N (Schering)
norethisterone
(progesterone hormone) | tablets | used to postpone menstruation and in the treatment of premenstrual syndrome, painful periods, heavy menstrual bleeding etc.

Primperan (Berk)
metoclopramide hydrochloride | tablets, medicine, injection | used in the treatment of stomach upsets of all kinds and to control nausea and vomiting

Prioderm (Napp)
malathion | skin preparation | used in the treatment of lice

With some drugs some side effects are common. But remember that all drugs may have any number of possible side effects; see p. 210

Pripsen (Reckitt & Colman) piperazine, sennoside	sachets	used in the treatment of worms
Pro-Actidil (Wellcome) triprolidine	tablets	used in the treatment of allergy problems; may cause drowsiness
probenecid†	tablets	used in the prevention of gout
Proctosedyl (Roussel) hydrocortisone (a steroid), cinchocaine, framycetin	skin preparation, suppositories	used in the treatment of hemorrhoids etc.
Progesic (Lilly) fenoprofen	tablets	a pain reliever
Progynova (Schering) oestradiol valerate	tablets	used in the treatment of menopause symptoms
promethazine†	tablets, medicine, injection	used in the treatment of allergies and the prevention of sickness; may cause drowsiness and dry mouth
Propaderm (A & H) beclomethazone dipropionate (a steroid)	skin preparation	used in the treatment of inflammatory skin conditions
Propain (Luitpold) paracetamol, codeine phosphate, diphenyramine hydrochloride, caffeine	tablets	a pain reliever
propranolol†	tablets, capsules, injections	used in the treatment of high blood pressure, angina, thyrotoxicosis; must not be stopped suddenly
Prothiaden (Boots) dothiepin	capsules, tablets	used in the treatment of depression
pyridostigmine†	tablets, injection	used in the treatment of myasthenia gravis
pyridoxine† (a member of the vitamin B group)	tablets	*see* p. 278
pyrimethamine†	tablets	an anti-malarial
Pyrogastrone (Winthrop) carbenoxolone, magnesium trisilicate, aluminium hydroxide	tablets	used in the treatment of ulcers etc.

Quellada (Stafford-Miller) gamma benzene hydrochloride	skin preparation	used in the treatment of scabies and body lice
quinidine†	tablets, capsules	used in the prevention and treatment of certain types of heartbeat irregularity
quinine†	tablets	used in the treatment of malaria; also in the prevention of night cramps
Quinoderm (Quinoderm) potassium hydroxyquinolone, sulphur, benzoyl peroxide	skin preparation	used in the treatment of acne etc.
Reactivan (Merck) fencamfamin hydrochloride, thiamine, pyridoxine, caynocobalamin, ascorbic acid	tablets	a stimulant
reserpine†	tablets	used in the treatment of high blood pressure; may cause dry mouth, sedation, depression
retinol† (vitamin A)	tablets, capsules	*see* p. 278
riboflavine† (a member of the vitamin B group)	tablets	*see* p. 278
rifampicin†	tablets, capsules, medicine	used in the treatment of tuberculosis
Rikospray (Riker) benzoin	aerosol	used to protect cracked nipples, bedsores etc.
Rinurel (Warner) paracetamol, phenylpropanolamine, phenyltolaxamine	tablets, medicine	used in the treatment of colds and flu; may cause drowsiness
Robitussin (Robins) guaiphenesin	medicine	used in the treatment of coughs
Ronicol (Roche) nicotinyl alcohol	tablets	used in the treatment of poor circulation

---

With some drugs some side effects are common. But remember that all drugs may have any number of possible side effects; see p. 210

Roter (FAIR) magnesium carbonate, bismuth subnitrate, sodium bicarbonate, frangula	tablets	an antacid
Rynacrom (Fisons) sodium cromoglycate	drops, spray, inhaler	used in the treatment of allergy states
Rythmodan (Roussel) disopyramide	tablets, capsules, injection	used in the prevention and control of irregular heartbeat
Safapryn (Pfizer) aspirin, paracetamol	tablets	a pain reliever
Safapryn Co (Pfizer) aspirin, paracetamol, codeine phosphate	tablets	a pain reliever
Salactol (Dermal) salicylic acid, lactic acid	skin preparation	used in the treatment of warts
salbutamol†	tablets, medicine, aerosol, injection	used in the treatment of bronchospasm (e.g. in asthma)
salicylic acid†	skin preparation	used in the treatment of warts
Saluric (MSD) chlorothiazide	tablets	a diuretic
Sando K (Sandoz) potassium bicarbonate, sodium saccharin, potassium chloride, docusate sodium	tablets	used in the prevention and treatment of potassium deficiency
Savlon (ICI) chlorhexidine gluconate	skin preparation	an anti-infective
Seconal (Lilly) quinalbarbitone (a barbiturate)	capsules	a hypnotic
Sectral (May & Baker) acebutolol hydrochloride	capsules, injection	used in the treatment of various heart conditions including angina and irregular heartbeat
selenium sulphide	skin preparation	used in the treatment of dandruff
Selsun (Abbott) selenium sulphide	skin preparation	used in the treatment of dandruff
senna†	tablets, granules, medicine	a laxative

Senokot (Reckitt & Colman) sennoside	tablets, granules, medicine	a laxative
Septrin (Wellcome) trimethoprim, sulphamethoxazole	tablets, medicine, injection	an anti-infective
Serenace (Searle) haloperidol	tablets, capsules, medicine, injection	used in the treatment of anxiety and a wide range of mental conditions
Serenid D (Wyeth) oxazepam (a benzodiazepine)	tablets, capsules	used in the treatment of anxiety etc.
Silbephylline (Berk) diprophylline	tablets, medicine, injection, suppositories	used in the treatment of bronchospasm (e.g. in asthma)
Sinemet (MSD) carbidopa, levodopa	tablets	used in the treatment of Parkinson's disease
Sinequan (Pfizer) doxepin hydrochloride	capsules	used in the treatment of anxiety and depression
Slow Fe (CIBA) ferrous sulphate	tablets	used in the prevention and treatment of iron deficiency anaemia
Slow K (CIBA) potassium chloride	tablets	used in the prevention and treatment of potassium deficiency; often prescribed in conjunction with diuretic therapy since some diuretics produce an excessive loss of potassium from the body
Slow Trasicor (CIBA) oxyprenolol	tablets	used in the treatment of heart conditions
smallpox vaccine†	injection	used to provide protection against smallpox (now extinct)
Sno-Phenicol Eye Drops (Smith & Nephew) chloramphenicol	eye drops	an anti-infective
sodium bicarbonate†	tablets, powder	an antacid; also used in replacement solution

---

With some drugs some side effects are common. But remember that all drugs may have any number of possible side effects; see p. 210

sodium cromoglycate†	inhaler, spray	used in the prevention of asthma
Solpadeine (Winthrop) paracetamol, codeine phosphate, caffeine	tablets	a pain reliever
Solprin (Reckitt & Colman) aspirin	tablets	a pain reliever
Sorbitrate (Stuart) isosorbide dinitrate	tablets	used in the prevention of angina
Sotacor (Bristol) sotalol	tablets, injection	used in the treatment of heart conditions
Sparine (Wyeth) promazine hydrochloride	tablets, injection, medicine	used in the treatment of agitation and many other mental conditions
Stelazine (Smith, Kline & French) trifluoperazine hydrochloride	tablets, capsules, medicine, injection	used in the treatment of anxiety and depression
Stemetil (May & Baker) prochlorperazine	tablets, medicine, suppositories, injection	used for numerous mental disorders but perhaps most widely prescribed to prevent nausea and vomiting
steroids *see* corticosteroids		
streptomycin†	injection	an anti-infective; used in the treatment of tuberculosis
Sudafed (Calmic) pseudoephedrine	tablets, medicine	used in the treatment of congestion
sulphacetamide†	eye ointment, drops	an anti-infective
sulphasalazine	tablets, suppositories	used in the control of inflammatory bowel conditions
Sultrin (Ortho) sulphathiazole, sulphacetamide, sulphabenzamide	skin preparation	an anti-infective
Surmontil (May & Baker) trimipramine maleate	tablets, capsules	used in the treatment of depression
Sustac (Pharmax) glyceryl trinitrate	tablets	used in the prevention of angina

Synalar (ICI) fluocinolone acetonide (a steroid)	skin preparation	used in the treatment of inflammatory skin conditions
Syntocinon (Sandoz) oxytocin (a hormone)	injection	stimulates the womb muscles; used to induce labour
Tagamet (Smith, Kline & French) cimetidine	tablets, injection	used in the treatment of peptic ulcers
Talpen (Beecham) talampicillin	tablets, medicine	an anti-infective
Tandacote (Geigy) oxyphenbutazone	tablets	used in the treatment of inflammatory conditions such as arthritis
Tanderil (Geigy) oxyphenbutazone	tablets, suppositories	used in the treatment of inflammatory conditions such as arthritis
Tedral (Warner) theophylline, ephedrine,	tablets, medicine	used in the treatment of inflammatory conditions such as arthritis
Tegretol (Geigy) carbamazepine	tablets, medicine	a pain reliever
Temgesic Sublingual (Reckitt & Colman) buprenorphine	tablets	a pain reliever
Tenormin (Stuart) atenolol	tablets	used in the treatment of heart disorders
Tenuate Dospan (Merrell) diethylpropion	tablets	used in the treatment of obesity
Teronac (Wander) mazindol	tablets	used in the treatment of obesity
Terramycin (Pfizer) oxytetracycline	capsules, medicine, injection	an anti-infective
testosterone† (a hormone)	tablets, injection, long-term implantation	male hormone replacement
tetanus vaccine†	injection	used to provide protection against tetanus

---

With some drugs some side effects are common. But remember that all
drugs may have any number of possible side effects; see p. 210

Tetrabid (Organon) tetracycline	capsules	an anti-infective
tetracycline†	tablets, medicine, injection	an anti-infective; not to be used by children under 12 because of adverse effect on developing teeth
Theocontin Continus (Napp) theophylline	tablets	used in the treatment of bronchospasm (e.g. in asthma)
thiamine† (a member of the vitamin B group)	tablets	*see* p. 278
Thovaline (Ilon) talc, kaolin, zinc oxide, cod liver oil, wool fat	skin preparation	used to soothe and protect inflamed or sore skin
thyroxin†	tablets	used in the treatment of hypothyroidism (thyroid deficiency)
timolol	tablets	a beta blocker; used in the treatment of angina and high blood pressure
Tinaderm (Kirby-Warrick) tolnaftate	skin preparation	used in the treatment of athlete's foot and similar conditions
Tineafax (Wellcome) zinc undecenoate	skin preparation	used in the treatment of athlete's foot and similar conditions
Tixylix (May & Baker) promethazine, pholcodine, phenylpropanolamine	medicine	used in the treatment of coughs; may cause drowsiness
Tofranil (Geigy) imipramine hydrochloride	tablets, medicine, injection	used in the treatment of depression and bed-wetting
Transvasin (Lloyds) tetra hydrofurfuryl salicylate, ethyl nicotinate, n-hexyl nicotinate, benzocaine	embrocation	used in the treatment of rheumatic ailments
Tranxene (Boehringer Ingelheim) potassium clorazepate (a benzodiazepine)	capsules	used in the treatment of anxiety; a single capsule is taken at night and is designed to have all-day action
Trasicor (CIBA) oxyprenolol	tablets, injection	used in the treatment of heart conditions

Trasidrex (CIBA)   tablets   used in the treatment of
oxyprenolol hydrochloride,   high blood pressure
cyclopenthiazide

Tri-Adcortyl (Squibb)   skin   used in the treatment of
(a steroid) triamcinolone   preparation   inflammatory skin conditions
acetonide, nystatin,   where infection is also
neomycin, gramicidin   suspected

Trilisate (Napp)   tablets   used in the treatment of
choline magnesium   rheumatoid arthritis,
trisalicylate   osteoarthritis etc.

Trimopan (Berk)   tablets   used as an anti-infective
trimethoprim

Trinordial (Wyeth)
oral contraceptive *see* p. 269

Tropium (DDSA)   tablets,   used in the treatment of
chlordiazepoxide   capsules   anxiety etc.
hydrochloride
(a benzodiazepine)

Tryptizol (Morson)   tablets,   used in the treatment of
amitriptyline hydrochloride   capsules,   depression and bed-wetting
                                        medicine

Tuinal (Lilly)   capsules   a hypnotic
quinalbarbitone,
amylobarbitone (barbiturates)

typhoid vaccine†   injection   used to provide protection
                                        against typhoid

Ultrabase (Schering)   skin   an emollient; plain cream
white soft paraffin, liquid   preparation   sometimes used as a base
paraffin, stearyl alcohol   for active preparations

Ultradil (Schering)   skin   used in the treatment of
fluocortolone pivalate,   preparation   inflammatory skin conditions
fluocortolone hexanoate
(steroids)

Ultralanum (Schering)   skin   used in the treatment of
fluocortolone (a steroid),   preparation   inflammatory skin conditions
clemizole, hexachlorophane   where an infection is
                                        present

With some drugs some side effects are common. But remember that all
drugs may have any number of possible side effects; see p. 210

Unguentum Merck (Merck) — skin preparation — an emollient; a plain cream sometimes used as a base for active preparations
silicic acid, liquid paraffin, white soft paraffin, cetostearyl alcohol, polysorbate 40, glycerol monostearate, saturated neutral oil, sorbic acid, propylene glycol

Urispas (Syntex) — tablets — used to control the bladder
flavoxate

Urolucosil (Warner) — tablets, medicine — an anti-infective
sulphamethizole

Uticillin (Beecham) — tablets — an anti-infective
carfecillin

Uvistat (WBP) — skin preparation — used to protect the skin from ultra-violet light
mexenone

vaccines *see* pp. 272 ff.

Valium (Roche) — tablets, capsules, medicine, injection — a tranquillizer used for a wide variety of conditions
diazepam (a benzodiazepine)

Vallergan (May & Baker) — tablets, medicine — used as a sedative and in the treatment of allergy problems; may cause drowsiness
trimeprazine

V-Cil-K (Lilly) — tablets, capsules, medicine — an anti-infective
penicillin V

Veganin (Warner) — tablets — a pain reliever
aspirin, paracetamol, codeine phosphate

Velosef (Squibb) — capsules, medicine, injection — an anti-infective
cephradine

Ventolin (A & H) — tablets, medicine, aerosol, injection — used in the treatment of bronchospasm (e.g. in asthma)
salbutamol

Veracur (Typharm) — skin preparation — used in the treatment of warts
formaldehyde

Vibramycin (Pfizer) — capsules, medicine — an anti-infective
doxycycline

Villescon (Boehringer Ingelheim) — medicine, tablets — a general tonic
prolintane, thiamine, riboflavine, pyridoxine, nicotinamide, ascorbic acid

Vioform (CIBA) clioquinol, hydrocortisone (a steroid)	skin preparation	used in the treatment of inflammatory skin conditions
Viskaldix (Sandoz) pindolol, clopamide	tablets	used in the treatment of high blood pressure
vitamins *see* p. 278		
Vivalan (ICI) viloxazine	tablets	an anti-depressant
Voltarol (Geigy) diclofenac	tablets, suppositories	used in the treatment of inflammatory diseases such as arthritis
warfarin†	tablets	an anti-coagulant; used in the treatment and prevention of blood clots
Waxsol (Norgine) docusate sodium	drops	used to help remove wax from the ears
Welldorm (Smith & Nephew) dichloralphenazone	tablets, medicine	a hypnotic
yellow fever vaccine†	injection	used to provide protection against yellow fever
Zaditen (Wander) ketotifen	tablets, capsules	used in the treatment of bronchospasm (e.g. in asthma)
Zomax (Ortho) zomepirac sodium	tablets	a pain reliever
Zyloric (Calmic) allopurinol	tablets	used in the treatment of gout

---

With some drugs some side effects are common. But remember that all drugs may have any number of possible side effects; see p. 210

Hormone treatments

A hormone is defined as a chemical substance produced in one organ within the body, carried in the blood stream and having an effect on other parts of the body. As the following list shows, hormones have a vital influence on the working of the human body. When hormone-producing organs fail to do their job properly the missing hormone can sometimes be replaced artificially with a specially prepared substitute. Sometimes these hormone substitutes can be given by mouth (for example, thyroxin) but sometimes they have to be given by injection (for example, insulin).

HORMONE	SECRETED BY	MAIN EFFECT
adrenaline	adrenal gland	stimulates heart and brain and prepares body for action
adrenocorticotropic hormone (ACTH)	pituitary gland	stimulates the adrenal gland
corticosteroids	adrenal gland	have a powerful effect on carbohydrate and protein metabolism, electrolyte balance and body's immune system
follicle stimulating hormone (FSH)	pituitary gland	stimulates production of eggs by ovary and sperm by testes
glucagon	pancreas	opposes effect of insulin
growth hormone	pituitary gland	governs growth of the body
insulin	pancreas	regulates use of sugar in body
noradrenalin	adrenal gland	constricts small arteries and has an effect on heart rate
oestrogen	ovaries	regulates development of female characteristics and menstrual cycle
oxytocin	neurohypophysis	stimulates womb muscles, fallopian tube contraction and production of milk by female breasts
parathyroid hormone	parathyroid gland	regulates calcium metabolism
progesterone	ovaries	works with oestrogen to control ovulation and pregnancy
prolactin	pituitary gland	regulates breast development and milk production
testosterone	testes	stimulates development of male characteristics
thyroid hormone	thyroid gland	regulates metabolism
thyroid stimulating hormone (TSH)	pituitary gland	stimulates thyroid gland

Oral contraceptives

Many millions of women have been using oral hormone preparations as contraceptives for a number of years now. There has inevitably been a great deal of research into the safety of these preparations and a large number of doctors and women consider that the risks, which undoubtedly exist, are acceptable. There are medical as well as social reasons for advocating the use of oral contraceptives rather than any other form of contraception, since the mortality and morbidity risks associated with abortions and pregnancy are thought to be much higher than those associated with the use of the contraceptive pill.

There are two main types of contraceptive pill available: the combination pills which contain a mixture of oestrogen and progesterone, and the progesterone-only pills. The combination pills are thought to be the most effective for general use and there is a wide range of such products on the market. The most important difference between the available products lies in the amount of oestrogen included in each pill. Generally speaking, those preparations that have the lowest oestrogen content are least effective if not taken regularly at the same time of day. Most doctors will, however, aim to find the pill with the lowest oestrogen content that properly controls the menstrual cycle, since the risks associated with taking the contraceptive pill increase with the level of oestrogen in the pill. The progesterone-only pills are usually prescribed for women who cannot take pills containing oestrogen, since they are usually less effective as contraceptives and there tends to be a greater risk of menstrual irregularity developing.

1   Oestrogen and progesterone contraceptives

(Combined oral contraceptives are usually classified according to the level of the oestrogen content.)

These contraceptives contain 50 micrograms of mestranol (an oestrogen):

Norinyl 1   Norinyl 1/28   Ortho-Novin 1/50

These contraceptives contain 50 micrograms of ethinyl-oestradiol (an oestrogen):

Anovlar 21	Minilyn	Orlest 21
Demulen 50	Minovlar	Ovran
Gynovlar 21	Norlestrin	Ovulen 50

These contraceptives contain 35 micrograms of ethinyl-oestradiol (an oestrogen):

Brevinor	Norimin	Ovysmen

These contraceptives contain 30 micrograms of ethinyl-oestradiol (an oestrogen):

Conova 30	Microgynon 30	Ovranette
Eugynon 30	Ovran 30	

This contraceptive contains 20 micrograms of ethinyloestradiol (an oestrogen):

Loestrin 20

2 Progesterone-only contraceptives

These contraceptives contain no oestrogen:

Femulen	Microval	Norgeston
Micronor	Neogest	Noriday

Using the contraceptive pill: points to remember

1 Contraceptive pills are extremely reliable if taken regularly. The manufacturer's instructions (usually included in each pack of pills) should be followed conscientiously and any warnings heeded.

2 Women who have a gastro-intestinal upset (vomiting or diarrhoea) while taking the pill should be aware that the effectiveness of the pill may be reduced, and women taking some other drugs (for example, some tranquillizers, pain relievers and antibiotics) should be aware that the effectiveness of the contraceptive pill may be diminished under these circumstances.

3 Most pills have to be taken for 21 days and then left alone for 7 days, but again the manufacturer's instructions should be followed.

4 Doctors vary in their attitudes towards the use of oral contraceptives directly following childbirth or during breastfeeding. Personally, I prefer women to have a normal period before starting the pill after the birth of a baby, and I will not prescribe the contraceptive pill to any woman who is breastfeeding. I appreciate that this is considered rather oldfashioned by a number of practitioners.

5 Many doctors believe that when possible oral contraceptives should not be taken in the month prior to surgery.

Side effects with oral contraceptives

All types of oral contraceptive can cause side effects. The ten commonest problems (in no particular order) are:

> nausea and vomiting
> headache
> breast tenderness
> changes in sexual activity and desire
> changes in body weight
> depression
> high blood pressure
> menstrual irregularity
> absence of periods
> acne and skin problems in general

Any one of these side effects can be dealt with by changing the pill (and therefore changing the proportion of oestrogen to progesterone). High menstrual loss, for example, can be reduced by using a pill with a high progesterone content, although this is likely to produce a greater increase in weight. It is wise to try a pill for three months before changing it since the body usually takes a month or two to settle.

The more serious side effects include blood clotting and heart troubles, and to avoid these problems it is wise to keep the oestrogen content as low as possible. Many doctors today feel that women who are overweight, who smoke, who are over the age of thirty-five, who have a family history of blood clots or diabetes, or who have high blood pressure should not be given the contraceptive pill, since the risk of clotting and heart disease rises in these circumstances.

Most doctors check the blood pressure of patients who are taking the contraceptive pill at least once a year.

Vaccines

Ten years ago smallpox affected millions of people around the world every year. Some died and others were scarred for life. Today, however, smallpox is officially extinct. There has not been a single case for over a year. The main reason that this once formidable killer disease has been tamed is the availability of an effective vaccine.

Similar, although less dramatic, stories can be told for other diseases such as poliomyelitis, diphtheria and tuberculosis. Vaccination has not been the only factor, but it has been a major one. Without effective vaccines all these diseases would still be largely untamed.

For two centuries now we have known that it is not necessary to suffer a disease in order to develop immunity to it. The human body can prepare the necessary defence mechanisms itself if given – by means of vaccination – what is effectively a very mild attack of the disease. Put very simply the body, when given a sneak preview of a potentially dangerous disease with its trousers down, can prepare suitable defence mechanisms which will provide protection against later exposure to the full power of the disease.

The extent of the protection that can be obtained and the time for which it will last obviously depends on the ease with which a suitable, effective vaccine can be prepared. For some diseases, such as polio and tetanus, available vaccines are effective and long lasting. For others, such as cholera, vaccines are not so effective nor so long lasting.

Even more important than the variation in the efficiency of the vaccines available is the risk of side effects occurring after vaccination. Any procedure which can save lives can also be hazardous and vaccination is no exception. The risks must always be weighed against the benefits.

In recent years the particular vaccine which has aroused most controversy has been the one used to protect against whooping cough (pertussis). A number of experts still claim that whooping cough vaccination is not only relatively inefficient but is also responsible for a relatively high number of problems. They say that there are, in particular, unacceptable risks of brain damage. Other experts, however, claim that the risks to the community of stopping whooping cough vaccination are greater than the risks of continuing. They argue that if no babies were vaccinated against whooping cough the incidence of the disease in the community would rise alarmingly.

Nevertheless, despite these reassurances a large number of parents have in recent years chosen not to have their babies vaccinated against whooping cough. Unhappily the use of other, safer vaccines has also suffered and some young children are now unprotected against tetanus, diphtheria and poliomyelitis.

In an attempt to clarify the situation regarding available vaccines I have in the rest of this section detailed the advantages and disadvantages of the commoner vaccines. I have listed the contra-indications to vaccination in an attempt to help readers decide when vaccination may or may not be suitable.

Since, however, vaccinations cannot be performed without a doctor's authorization it is important to discuss the suitability of a specific vaccine with the doctor concerned. You should make available any relevant medical information if the doctor is not your usual general practitioner. If you are not sure whether or not specific information is relevant then you should mention it anyway.

When to be vaccinated

All vaccinations except for polio are generally given by injection; polio is usually given orally.

Vaccinations can be combined, and there are several double and triple vaccines. Diphtheria can be combined with tetanus, and typhoid with paratyphoid. Diphtheria, tetanus and pertussis; typhoid, paratyphoid A and B and tetanus; and typhoid, paratyphoid A and B and cholera are often given as triple vaccines. (In some areas vaccination schedules may differ from those given below.)

cholera
If you are travelling to Africa, the Middle East or the Far East, and occasionally if you are travelling to a Mediterranean country (check with your travel agent), you should be vaccinated against cholera. It is inadvisable for young children to have a cholera vaccination.

diphtheria
Children should be vaccinated against diphtheria at the age of three months, and then again at six and twelve months. The vaccination is usually combined with the tetanus vaccination. People over the age of ten years who have not been vaccinated need to be tested for immunity before vaccination. There are no known circumstances where the diphtheria vaccination must be avoided.

infective hepatitis
If you intend to live rough in a Third World country it may be worth asking your doctor to consider giving you a protective injection of immuno-globulin.

influenza
This vaccination is usually only given to adults at risk (such as sufferers of chronic bronchitis who would be in danger if they contracted flu). Influenza vaccination is avoided if the individual is allergic to eggs (*see* measles), and should only be given to children under the age of nine years if they are suffering from a chronic lung or heart disease. In such cases, a reduced dose of the vaccine is essential.

measles
The measles vaccination is given to children in their second or third year. Vaccination is avoided if there is any history of fits, epilepsy or convulsions associated either with the child concerned or with his or her family. It should be avoided if there are any signs of physical under-development, and if there is an allergy to the antibiotics neomycin or polymyxin (rarely prescribed), or to eggs (patients allergic to eggs develop general 'allergy' symptoms such as rashes, wheezes or vomiting). If these contra-indications are ignored, reactions of various kinds can occur, convulsions being the most potentially serious.

poliomyelitis

All children should be vaccinated against polio at the age of three months and again at the ages of six and twelve months. An oral vaccine is usually given at the same time as the diphtheria and tetanus injection. Children should then be re-vaccinated at the age of six years, and on leaving school. Frequent travellers abroad should have booster doses every three years. Polio vaccination is avoided if there is diarrhoea and/or vomiting (to ensure full protection the symptoms must have subsided), or if there is any allergy to the antibiotics neomycin or polymyxin (rarely prescribed) or streptomycin.

rubella (German measles)

Girls should be vaccinated at the age of eleven whether or not they are thought to have had the disease, as diagnosis is often difficult. Vaccination is avoided during pregnancy, and pregnancy should be avoided for three months after vaccination. (Pregnant women given the vaccine can produce deformed babies.) At least one month should elapse between rubella and TB injections. Patients allergic to rabbits, neomycin and polymyxin should avoid the vaccination.

smallpox

Vaccination against smallpox is now unnecessary as the disease is officially extinct. If you are going abroad some countries will still ask for a certificate of vaccination but should be satisfied with a letter from your doctor.

tetanus

All children should be vaccinated at the age of three months and then again at six and twelve months; usually the vaccine is given along with the diphtheria and polio vaccines. A booster should be given when the child reaches the age of six and another when he or she leaves school. People liable to sustain dirty wounds (e.g. farmers, gardeners, soccer players) should have boosters every three years; otherwise boosters are only necessary on injury. You should not have more than one booster in any one year. If the vaccine is given too frequently, there can be a reaction with a painful red swelling appearing at the injection site.

tuberculosis

At the age of eleven all children should be tested for TB immunity and if the reaction is negative they should be vaccinated (the vaccine is known as BCG). The disease is still prevalent in immigrant areas. Vaccination is avoided in cases of eczema or of local skin infections. The rubella (German measles) vaccination should be avoided for one month, and all other injections in the same arm for three months, after the TB vaccination.

typhoid

The typhoid vaccination is usually given with paratyphoid A and B. Travellers to most countries outside northern Europe and North America should be vaccinated; regular travellers should have vaccinations every three years. It is inadvisable for young children to have a typhoid vaccination.

whooping cough (pertussis)
Whooping cough vaccination is usually given at three, six and twelve months along with diphtheria and tetanus. Whooping cough is the least effective of these three and some experts believe that there are serious risks involved in giving the vaccination (see p. 273). If there are doubts, the vaccination may be omitted. The vaccination is avoided if there is any history of fits, epilepsy or convulsions associated either with the child concerned or with his or her family. Similarly if there is any history of allergy (eczema, asthma, hay fever), or if the child's birth was difficult, vaccination should be avoided. There is a risk of brain damage if these contra-indications are ignored. If there is any severe local or general reaction to the first injection, further injections are probably best avoided.

yellow fever
Travellers to central Africa and Central and South America should be vaccinated against yellow fever. Infants under the age of nine months should not have the vaccination, and it should not be given to people allergic to eggs (*see* measles) or to neomycin and polymyxin.

Vitamins

Vitamins are essential nutrients about which we still know remarkably little, apart from the fact that a well-balanced diet is one that will contain enough vitamins to satisfy the body's requirements. Extra vitamins are potentially dangerous and will do the body no good at all unless there is an existing deficiency. Trying to become fitter by taking extra vitamins is as logical as trying to make a motor car go faster by struggling to pump 1000 gallons of petrol into the tank or trying to get a better TV picture by putting 500,000 volts into the TV set.

When vitamins were first discovered at the beginning of the 20th century they were given letters as they were identified. Soon after the first vitamins had been labelled, it was discovered that the substance called vitamin B actually consisted of several different substances, and scientists then had to name the vitamins in the B group B_1, B_2, B_3 and so on all the way up to vitamin B_{12}.

Later still it was discovered that vitamins such as B_3, B_5 and B_7 were not, after all, separate vitamins. And so the B group of vitamins now simply consists of vitamin B_1, B_2, B_4, B_6 and B_{12}. To add to the confusion the vitamins in this group are also given names: vitamin B_1 is also known as aneurine or thiamine; B_2 is known as riboflavine; B_6 is called pyridoxine; and B_{12} is cyanocobalamin. Vitamin C, by the way, is known as ascorbic acid.

As I have already pointed out we are still very ignorant about vitamins but we do know that vitamin A is needed to help keep the skin and eyes healthy; that vitamin B helps the body make proper use of foodstuffs; that vitamin C is needed for the development and maintenance of body tissues; and that vitamin D is vital to help the body turn calcium into bone.

It is easy to ensure that the body is kept well supplied with all these essential nutrients. Vitamin A is present in milk, eggs, butter, cheese, liver and fish oils and in those vegetables (such as carrots) which contain carotene. Vitamin B is found in a wide range of animal and vegetable products. Vitamin C is found in fruit and vegetables. Vitamin D is present in cheese, butter, margarine, fish and animal livers and oils. There is also enough sunshine in most countries in the world to provide the majority of people with a good proportion of the vitamin D they need.

It is clear, then, that a diet which includes meat, fish or eggs; fruit or vegetables; milk or cheese; margarine or butter and some cereals will provide a good assortment of essential vitamins.

Taking extra vitamins, on the other hand, can be dangerous and even fatal, and no one should ever take supplementary vitamins which have not been prescribed by a doctor.

A to Z glossary of pharmaceutical terms

aerosol
Solid or liquid particles of medicament suspended in a fine spray or mist.

anaesthetic
A product that dulls the senses. In home use, this invariably means a cream or spray which helps control irritation or pain.

analgesic
A pain reliever

anorectic
A drug that reduces the appetite. Clearly most slimming drugs fall into this category.

antacid
Something that counteracts or opposes the action of an acid. Antacids are usually prescribed for the relief of indigestion pains which may be exacerbated by the excessive production or availability of stomach acid.

antibiotic
A chemical product which destroys living organisms. Antibiotics intended for use by mouth usually have to be prescribed by a doctor but there are creams, ointments and so on containing antibiotics which are available for home use.

anticholinergic
A drug which interferes with the process whereby nervous impulses are passed through the body. It is sometimes used in the prevention of motion sickness, for example.

anti-emetic
A product designed to prevent vomiting.

antihistamine
A substance which counteracts the effects of 'histamine', a chemical which is released within the body automatically when tissues are injured but which itself has unwanted effects. Reddening of the skin which occurs after a sting is caused by the production of histamine. An antihistamine drug can prevent that reaction developing.

anti-infective
I have used this term widely in this book to describe all groups of drugs used in the treatment of infection. Some anti-infective drugs are only effective against bacteria while others are, for example, only effective against fungal infections.

anti-inflammatory
A drug which helps oppose inflammatory processes within the body. Inflammation can be caused by injury or infection and usually involves heat, redness, swelling and pain. An anti-inflammatory drug can help control those symptoms.

antiperspirant
A product which prevents sweating, for example by blocking the pores in the skin.

antipyretic
Something which helps bring down a fever or temperature. Aspirin, for example, has an antipyretic action.

antiseptic
A substance which destroys small organisms that may harm living tissue (*see* disinfectant).

antispasmodic
A drug which helps stop spasms. Muscle spasms can be a cause of pain, and an antispasmodic may therefore effectively prevent or relieve pain.

anxiolytic
A drug designed to help an anxious or worried patient. Effective anxiolytics usually need to be obtained on prescription.

aperient
A gentle laxative or fairly mild 'opening' medicine.

application
Any liquid or semi-liquid preparation which is applied to the skin.

astringent
Strictly speaking an astringent is something that prevents a discharge of any kind. Substances which stop bleeding may be astringents.

balm
An aromatic ointment that is used to help heal a wound or to soothe pain. Balms are commonly used in the treatment of rheumatism.

cachet
A wafer or capsule which contains a medicinal substance.

capsule
A small soluble container which dissolves in the body releasing the medicine that is contained within it – usually in powder form. The two halves of a capsule are often coloured separately.

cathartic
A purgative or laxative. Something which helps to empty the bowels.

caustic
A substance which can burn and destroy.

collodion
A clear sticky liquid used to hold wounded edges together, hold dressings in place and seal sterile wounds. If medicaments are dissolved in a collodion their contact with the skin is prolonged.

cough suppressant
A substance which helps a patient actually stop coughing. Some cough medicines are not, in fact, designed to do this (*see* expectorant).

cream
A medical substance with the consistency of the top of the milk. Creams spread more easily than ointments which tend to be stickier.

decongestant
Usually means something which helps to relieve congestion or stuffiness in the nose and sinuses.

deodorant
A product designed to remove (or prevent) unwanted body smells. A deodorant may contain a disinfectant (intended to destroy organisms which might otherwise break down human sweat and in the process produce a nasty smell), and/or a perfume designed simply to disguise unpleasant smells.

disinfectant
A substance which destroys the small organisms that may produce infection and harm living tissue. The word 'disinfectant' is usually kept for products which are used on inanimate objects which need to be kept clean (dirty sheets may be washed in a disinfectant), whereas the word 'antiseptic' is usually kept for products used on the human body (mouthwashes, lotions, creams and so on). However, this distinction is not always followed and the two words are often used as though they were interchangeable. Just to make matters even more confused there are manufacturers who claim that their products contain antiseptics and disinfectants. But, essentially, the words antiseptic and disinfectant do mean the same thing.

diuretic
A product which increases the flow of urine. By increasing the rate at which water is excreted from the body a diuretic may help reduce ankle swelling or other signs of fluid retention.

dusting powder
A fine powder which is shaken onto the body like talcum powder.

elixir
A sweetened aromatic preparation of a soluble medicinal substance. Elixirs are given 'miracle' properties by those with an interest in their sale.

embrocation
A liquid rubbed onto the affected part of the body to ease pain.

emollient
An application rubbed onto the body to help soften and relax it.

emulsion
A mixture of two immiscible liquids, one dispersed throughout the other in small droplets.

enema
A solution designed for introduction into the rectum, either to promote evacuation of the bowel contents or to introduce food, medicine or X-ray material.

expectorant
A medicine which helps a patient bring up sputum. It works by liquefying secretions which already exist or by encouraging the production of fluids which will dilute secretions.

gargle
A solution for rinsing mouth and throat.

gel
A jelly-like material.

germicide
An agent that destroys small organisms. For practical purposes, the term germicide is interchangeable with antiseptic and disinfectant.

granules
Medicinal pellets which may be taken with or without water.

hypnotic
A drug that helps produce sleep. Powerful hypnotics are only available on prescription and mild hypnotics probably rely heavily on the placebo effect (see p. 200).

inhalation
A preparation designed to be drawn into the lungs. If you fill a bowl with hot water, cover your head with a towel and breathe in the steam rising from the bowl through your nostrils you are inhaling water vapour. (This can help catarrh etc.)

injection
The introduction of a liquid into the body. Injections can be into muscles, tissues or directly into blood vessels. Strictly speaking an enema is inserted by injection.

insufflation
A powder, vapour or gas designed to be blown into a body cavity – for example the mouth and throat. Problems can occur if the patient blows back!

keratolytic
A powerful substance used to destroy unwanted skin (such as warts and corns) but which can damage good, healthy skin.

laxative
A medicine which helps empty the bowels. Laxative, purgative and cathartic all mean the same thing.

linctus
A syrupy medicine designed to be licked up with the tongue.

liniment
An oily liquid preparation to be rubbed onto the skin.

lotion
A liquid preparation for bathing a part of the body.

lozenge
A medicated troche. A troche is a dry, solid, medicated mass intended to be held in the mouth and slowly dissolved in the saliva. It was originally diamond-shaped.

medicated
This word is used by many manufacturers as though it automatically improved the quality of any product. It simply means that the product concerned in some way contains a substance which has medicinal properties. For example, sticking plasters treated with antiseptics are described as 'medicated', as are sweets containing minute quantities of substances which have mild medicinal qualities.

mixture
A medicinal preparation of two or more ingredients mixed together. Some manufacturers put dozens of different ingredients into their mixtures but frequently none of the ingredients are included in worthwhile quantities.

mouthwash
see gargle.

ointment
A semi-solid preparation for external application to the body maybe containing a medicinal substance such as an antihistamine or an antibiotic. Ointments are greasier, stickier and messier than creams but can be useful on very dry, crusty skin.

paint
An external medicament which is put on with a brush – like any other paint!

paste
A semi-solid preparation, usually applied to the skin. Pastes are firmer than ointments.

pessary
An instrument placed inside the vagina to support the uterus, or a medicated vaginal suppository.

pill
A convenient way to serve up small doses of medicine in a suitable size for swallowing. Pills were originally prepared by hand – the chemist rolling the substances between his fingers with the movement that people use when playing with small pieces of bread or plasticine.

potion
A large dose of liquid medicine – one that needs to be drunk rather than simply taken on a spoon.

poultice
A soft pulpy mass placed hot upon the skin as a counter-irritant to soothe a sore or inflamed part of the body. A hot-water bottle is probably just as good but is nowhere near as much fun.

powder
A lot of tiny particles obtained by grinding a solid mass. Chemists used to use a mortar and pestle to make powders (the mortar is the bowl).

preservative
Labels on medicine bottles often list ingredients described as preservatives. These substances do exactly the same job as the preservatives added to foodstuffs – they help to stop the product going bad.

prophylactic

Strictly speaking a prophylactic is anything which helps prevent disease. In everyday language, however, a prophylactic often means a condom. This specialized definition has some validity if you regard pregnancy as a disease.

purgative

A medicine which helps empty the bowels (*see* laxative). The British sometimes seem to be obsessed with the behaviour of their bowels and the number of available words which can be used to describe drugs which have an effect on 'stubborn' bowels illustrates this obsession rather well.

rub

A substance suitable for rubbing onto the skin (*see* liniment *and* rubefacient).

rubefacient

A substance that reddens and irritates the skin.

sedative

A drug which has a calming effect. Most sedatives also cause drowsiness. Powerful sedatives are only available on prescription.

shake lotions

A convenient way of applying powder to the skin. The water in which the powder is suspended evaporates, cooling and soothing the skin, and leaves the powder behind. Obviously needs to be shaken before use. Calamine lotion is a good example.

solution

An evenly distributed solid available in liquid form.

spirit

A volatile or distilled liquid.

spray

A liquid which is available as a mist — a lot of tiny droplets.

stimulant

A substance which excites all or part of the human body. Caffeine is a stimulant which has a general effect on human beings.

suppository

A medicated solid mass of suitable size and consistency for inserting into a body cavity other than the mouth, e.g. the vagina, the rectum or the urethra. Pessaries are suppositories which are placed inside the vagina.

tablet

A small amount of a drug compressed or moulded into shape by machine and containing a fixed amount of active ingredients. A tablet may be coated with various substances to conceal the taste or to delay its disintegration and absorption. Most modern pills are in fact tablets.

tranquillizer

A medicine which has a calming effect. Tranquillizers are supposed to cause less drowsiness than sedatives but in practical terms this difference is usually rather slight.

vapour rub

A substance for rubbing onto the skin which gives off a vapour and smells medicinal.

vasodilator

A chemical which opens up the blood vessels and thereby encourages the flow of blood to the tissues. Products designed for use by patients with chilblains may be described as vasodilators. There is much contradictory evidence about the effectiveness of drugs in this category.

A to Z directory of major UK drug companies

Abbott Laboratories Ltd
Queenborough, Kent ME11 5EL

Alcan Laboratories (UK) Ltd
Imperial Way, Watford, Herts WD2 4YR

Alembic
Oaklands Drive, Sale, Manchester M33 1WS

Allen & Hanburys Ltd
Bethnal Green, London E2 6LA

Allergan Ltd
Bourne House, Wharf Lane, Bourne End, Bucks HP11 1JT

American Critical Care (formerly known as Arnar-Stone Laboratories)
Division of American Hospital Supply (UK) Ltd, Tileman House, 131 Upper
Richmond Road, London SW15 2TR

American Hospital Supply (UK) Ltd
131 Upper Richmond Road, London SW15 2TR

Ames Co. Ltd *see* Dome Division

Approved Prescription Services Ltd
Whitcliffe House, Whitcliffe Road, Cleckheaton, West Yorks BD19 3BZ

Armour Pharmaceutical Co. Ltd
Hampden Park, Eastbourne, East Sussex BN22 9AG

Associated Hospital Supply
PO Box 4, Pershore, Worcs WR10 1AJ

Astra Pharmaceuticals Ltd
St Peter's House, 2 Bricket Road, St Albans, Herts AL1 3JW

Ayerst Laboratories Ltd
Invincible Road, Farnborough, Hants GU14 7QH

C. R. Bard Int. Ltd
Pennywell Industrial Estate, Sunderland SR4 9EW

Bayer UK Ltd
Pharmaceutical Division, Burrell Road, Haywards Heath, West
Sussex RH16 1TP

BDH Pharmaceuticals Ltd
Lenten House, Lenten Street, Alton, Hants GU34 1JD

Beecham Research Laboratories
Great West Road, Brentford, Middlesex TW8 9BD

Bencard
PO Box 20, Brentford, Middlesex TW8 9BE

Bengue & Co. Ltd
St Ives House, St Ives Road, Maidenhead, Berks SL6 1RD

Berk Pharmaceuticals Ltd
Station Road, Shalford, Guildford, Surrey GU14 8HE

Bioglan Laboratories Ltd
Spirella Building, Bridge Road, Letchworth, Herts SG6 4ET

Boehringer Ingelheim Ltd
Southern Industrial Estate, Bracknell, Berks RG12 4YS

The Boots Company Ltd
1 Thane Road West, Nottingham NG2 3AA

Bristol Laboratories (division of Bristol-Myers Co. Ltd)
Station Road, Langley, Slough, Berks SL3 6EB

British Surgical Houses Ltd
3 Miles Buildings, Bath, Avon BA1 2QS

Brocades (Great Britain) Ltd
Brocades House, Pyrford Road, West Byfleet, Weybridge, Surrey KT14 6RA

Edwin Burgess Ltd
Longwick Road, Princes Risborough, Aylesbury, Bucks HP17 9RR

Calmic Medical Division
The Wellcome Foundation Ltd, Crewe Hall, Crewe, Cheshire CW1 1UB

Cambmac Instruments Ltd
Cambridge Road, Milton, Cambridge CB4 4AZ

The Cantassium Company
Larkhall Laboratories, 225 Putney Bridge Road, London SW15 2PY

Carnegie Medical
1 Morley Street, Loughborough, Leics LE11 1EP

Carnrick Laboratories (division of G. W. Carnrick Co. Ltd)
Victoria House, Vernon Place, Southampton Row, London WC1B 4EA

Carter-Wallace Ltd
Wear Bay Road, Folkstone, Kent CT19 6PG

CIBA Laboratories
Wimblehurst Road, Horsham, West Sussex RH12 4AB

Coates and Cooper Ltd (member of Napp Pharmaceutical Group)
Hill Farm Avenue, Watford, Herts WD2 7RA

L. D. Collins & Co. Ltd
49 High Street, Barnet, Herts EN5 5UW

Coloplast Ltd
Somersham Road, St Ives, Huntingdon, Cambs PE17 4LN

Comprehensive Pharmaceuticals Ltd
95 Frampton Street, London NW8 8NA

Concept Pharmaceuticals Ltd
Russell House, 59–61 High Street, Rickmansworth, Herts WD3 1EZ

Consolidated Chemicals Ltd
The Industrial Estate, Wrexham, Clwyd LL13 9PS, Wales

Cooper Health Products Ltd
Gatehouse Road, Aylesbury, Bucks HP19 3ED

Cow & Gate Ltd
Trowbridge, Wilts BA14 8HZ

Cox-Continental Ltd
Brookside Avenue, Rustington, West Sussex BN16 3LF

The Crookes Laboratories Ltd
Telford Road, Basingstoke, Hants RG21 2XZ

Dales Pharmaceuticals Ltd
Barrows Lane, Steeton, Keighley, West Yorks BD20 6PP

Davis-Geck (division of Cyanamid of Great Britain Ltd)
Fareham Road, Gosport, Hants PO13 0AS

DDSA Pharmaceuticals Ltd
310 Old Brompton Road, London SW5 9JQ

Delandale Laboratories Ltd
Delandale House, 37 Old Dover Road, Canterbury, Kent CT1 3JB

Dermal Laboratories Ltd
Tatmore Place, Gosmore, Hitchin, Herts SG4 7QR

Dermalex Co. Ltd
146–154 Kilburn High Road, London NW6 4JD

E. C. De Witt & Co. Ltd
Seymour Road, Leyton, London E10 7LX

Dista Products Ltd
Kingsclere Road, Basingstoke, Hants RG21 2XA

Dome Division
Miles Laboratories Ltd, Stoke Court, Stoke Poges, Slough, Berks SL2 4LY

Downs Surgical Ltd
Church Path, Mitcham, Surrey CR4 3UE

Duncan, Flockhart & Co. Ltd
Birkbeck Street, London E2 6LA

Duphar Laboratories Ltd
Gaters Hill, West End, Southampton SO3 3JD

Eaton Laboratories
Regent House, The Broadway, Woking, Surrey GU21 5AP

Ethicon Ltd
PO Box 408, Bankhead Avenue, Edinburgh EH11 4HE

Evans Medical Ltd
891–995 Greenford Road, Greenford, Middlesex UB6 0HE

FAIR Laboratories Ltd
179 Heath Road, Twickenham, Middlesex TW1 4BJ

Farillon Ltd
Bryant Avenue, Romford, Essex RM3 0PJ

Farley Health Products Ltd
Torr Lane, Plymouth, Devon PL3 5UA

Farmitalia Carlo Erba Ltd
Kingmaker House, Station Road, Barnet, Herts EN5 1NU

Ferring Pharmaceuticals Ltd
7 York Street, Twickenham, Middlesex TW1 3JZ

Fisons Ltd
Pharmaceutical Division, 12 Derby Road, Loughborough, Leics LE11 0BB

G. F. Dietary Supplies Ltd
7 Queensbury Station Parade, Queensbury, Edgware, Middlesex HA8 5NP

Galen Ltd
19 Lower Seagoe Industrial Estate, Portadown, Craigavon,
Co. Armagh BT63 5QD

Geigy Pharmaceuticals
Wimblehurst Road, Horsham, West Sussex RH12 4AB

Geistlich Sons Ltd
Newton Bank, Long Lane, Chester CH2 3QZ

Glaxo Laboratories Ltd
891–995 Greenford Road, Greenford, Middlesex UB6 0HE

Glenwood Laboratories Ltd
19 Wincheap, Canterbury, Kent CT1 3TB

Thomas Glover & Son Ltd
Carlton, Nottingham NG4 1EG

Hoechst UK Ltd
Pharmaceutical Division, Hoechst House, Salisbury Road, Hounslow,
Middlesex TW4 6JH

Hough, Houseason & Co. Ltd
22 Chapel Street, Levenshulme, Manchester M19 3PT

Immuno Ltd
Arctic House, Rye Lane, Dunton Green, Nr Sevenoaks, Kent TN14 5HB

Imperial Chemical Industries (ICI)
Pharmaceuticals Division, Alderley House, Alderley Park, Macclesfield,
Cheshire SK10 4TF

Ilon Laboratories Ltd
Lorne Street, Hamilton, Lanarks ML3 9AB

Innoxa Ltd
202 Terminus Road, Eastbourne, Sussex BN21 3DF

International Laboratories Ltd
Charwell House, Wilsom Road, Alton, Hants GU34 2TJ

Ernest Jackson & Co. Ltd
High Street, Crediton, Devon EX17 3AP

Janssen Pharmaceutical Ltd
Janssen House, Chapel Street, Marlow, Bucks SL7 1ET

Johnson & Johnson Ltd
260 Bath Road, Slough, Berks SL1 4EA

KabiVitrum Ltd
Bilton House, 54–58 Uxbridge Road, Ealing, London W5 2TH

Keeler Optical Products Ltd
Clewer Hill Road, Windsor, Berks SL4 4AA

Keymer *see* Schering Chemicals

Kirby-Warrick Pharmaceuticals
Mildenhall, Bury St Edmunds, Suffolk IP28 7AX

Labaz
Heaton Lane, Stockport, Cheshire SK4 1AG

Laboratories for Applied Biology Ltd
91 Amhurst Park, London N16 5DR

Lamberts (Dalston) Ltd
PO Box 136, 200 Queensbridge Road, London E8 3LY

Larkhall Laboratories
225 Putney Bridge Road, London SW15 2PY

Lastonet Products Ltd
Carn Brea, Redruth, Cornwall TR15 3QN

Lederle Laboratories
Fareham Road, Gosport, Hants PO13 0AS

Lenton Products
Castle Boulevard, Nottingham N67 1HF

Leo Laboratories Ltd
Longwick Road, Princes Risborough, Aylesbury, Bucks HP17 9RR

Lepetit Pharmaceuticals Ltd
Meadowbank, Bath Road, Hounslow, Middlesex TW5 9QY

Lewis Laboratories Ltd
Lavender Walk, Leeds LS9 8JG

Eli Lilly & Co. Ltd
Kingsclere Road, Basingstoke, Hants RG21 2XA

Lipha Pharmaceuticals Ltd
Old Farm Road, West Drayton, Middlesex UB7 7LD

Lloyd Anpher Ltd
Reckitt & Colman, Pharmaceutical Division, Dansom Lane, Hull HU8 7DS

Lloyd-Hamol Ltd
Reckitt & Colman, Pharmaceutical Division, Dansom Lane, Hull HU8 7DS

F. Longdon & Co. Ltd
Agard Street, Derby DE1 1EB

J. M. Loveridge Ltd
6 Millbrook Road, Southampton, Hants SO9 3LT

Loxley Medical
Bessinby Estate, Bridlington, N. Humberside YO16 4SU

LRC Products Ltd
North Circular Road, Chingford, London E4 8QA

Luitpold-Werk (Munich) (medical & scientific office in UK)
Hayes Gate House, 27 Uxbridge Road, Hayes, Middlesex UB4 0JD

Lundbeck Ltd
Lundbeck House, Hastings Street, Luton, Beds LU1 5BE

3M United Kingdom Ltd
PO Box 1, Bracknell, Berks RG12 1JU

Maltown Ltd
PO Box 53, Harrogate, North Yorks HG2 0NH

May & Baker Ltd
Rainham Road South, Dagenham, Essex RM10 7XS

MCP Pharmaceuticals Ltd
Grange Road, Houston Industrial Estate, Livingston, West Lothian EH54 5DE

Mead Johnson (division of Bristol-Myers Co. Ltd)
Station Road, Langley, Slough, Berks SL3 0ED

Medexport Ltd
76 Wells Street, London W1P 3RE

Medo-Chemicals Ltd
The Limes, 30 High Street, Chesham, Bucks HP5 1EP

E. Merck Ltd
Winchester Road, Four Marks, Alton, Hants GU34 5HG

Merck Sharp & Dohme Ltd
Hertford Road, Hoddesdon, Herts EN11 9BU

Merrell Division
Richardson-Merrell Ltd, 20 Queensmere, Slough, Berks SL1 1YY

Montedison Pharmaceuticals Ltd *see* Farmitalia Carlo Erba Ltd

Thomas Morson Pharmaceuticals
Hertford Road, Hoddesdon, Herts EN11 9BU

Napp Laboratories Ltd
Hill Farm Avenue, Watford, Herts WD2 7RA

Nestle Company Ltd
St George's House, Croydon, Surrey CR9 1NR

Nicholas Laboratories Ltd
PO Box 17, Slough, Berks SL1 4AU

Norgine Ltd
59–62 High Holborn, London WC1V 6EB

Norma Chemicals Ltd *see* Wallace

H. N. Norton & Co. Ltd
133a Shawbridge Street, Glasgow G43 1QQ

Novo Laboratories Ltd
Ringway House, Bell Road, Daneshill East, Basingstoke, Hants RG24 0QN

Organon Laboratories Ltd
Crown House, London Road, Morden, Surrey SM4 5DZ

Organon Teknika Ltd
Teknika House, Cromwell Road, St Neots, Huntingdon, Cambs PE19 2HS

Ortho Pharmaceutical Ltd
PO Box 79, Saunderton, High Wycombe, Bucks HP14 4HJ

Paines & Byrne Ltd
Pabyrn Laboratories, Bilton Road, Perivale, Greenford, Middlesex UB6 7HG

Parke, Davis & Company
Usk Road, Pontypool, Gwent NP4 0YH

Pettibone UK Ltd
Norton Street, Manchester M10 8AD

Pfizer Ltd
Sandwich, Kent CT13 9NJ

Pharmaceutical Manufacturing Co
Westhoughton, Bolton, Lancs BL5 3SL

Pharmacia (Great Britain) Ltd
Prince Regent Road, Hounslow, Middlesex TW3 1NE

Pharmax Ltd
Bourne Road, Bexley, Kent DA5 1NX

Phillips Yeast Products Ltd
47 Park Royal Road, London NW10 7JX

Plough (UK) Ltd
Penarth Street, Peckham, London SE15 1TT

Potter & Clarke Ltd
415 Limpsfield Road, Warlingham, Surrey CR3 9YS

Prentif (Surgical) Ltd *see* Lamberts

Priory Laboratories Ltd
Hill Farm Avenue, Watford, Herts WD2 7RA

Procea
Alexandra Road, Dublin

Quinoderm Ltd
Manchester Road, Hollinwood, Oldham, Lancs OL8 4PB

Radiol Chemicals Ltd
Stepfield, Witham, Essex, CM8 3AG

Raymed
Viaduct Road, Leeds LS4 2BR

Reckitt & Colman Pharmaceutical Division
Dansom Lane, Hull HU8 7DS

Reckitt-Labaz
Dansom Lane, Hull HU8 7DS

W. J. Rendell Ltd
Ickleford Manor, Hitchin, Herts SG5 3XE

Riker Laboratories
Morley Street, Loughborough, Leics LE11 1EP

Rimmer Bros
18–19 Aylesbury Street, London EC1R 0DD

A. H. Robins Co. Ltd
Redkiln Way, Horsham, West Sussex RH13 5QP

Robinson & Sons Ltd
Wheat Bridge, Chesterfield, Derbyshire S40 2AD

Roche Products Ltd
PO Box 8, Welwyn Garden City, Herts AL7 3AY

Rona Laboratories Ltd
Cadwell Lane, Hitchin, Herts SG4 0SF

Roussel Laboratories Ltd
Roussel House, North End Road, Wembley Park, Middlesex HA9 0NF

Roussel Medical Ltd
Delves Road, Heanor Gate, Heanor, Derbyshire DE7 7SJ

Rybar Laboratories Ltd
St Ives House, St Ives Road, Maidenhead, Berks SL6 1RD

E. Sallis Ltd
Vernon Works, Basford, Nottingham NG6 0DH

Salt & Son Ltd
220 Corporation Street, Birmingham B4 6QR

SAS Scientific Chemicals Ltd
Victoria House, Vernon Place, London WC1B 4DF

Sandoz Products Ltd
Sandoz House, 98 The Centre, Feltham, Middlesex TW13 4EP

Schering Chemicals Ltd
Pharmaceutical Division, Burgess Hill, West Sussex RH15 9NE

Scholl UK Ltd
182–204 St John Street, London EC1P 1DH

Scientific Hospital Supplies Ltd
38 Queensland Street, Liverpool L7 3JG

Searle Pharmaceutical Products Ltd
PO Box 53, Lane End Road, High Wycombe, Bucks HP12 4HI

Serono Laboratories (UK) Ltd
2 Tewin Court, Welwyn Garden City, Hereford AL7 1AU

Servier Laboratories Ltd
Servier House, Horsenden Lane South, Greenford, Middlesex UB6 7PW

Seton Products Ltd
Medlock Street, Oldham, Lancs OL1 3HS

Simpla Plastics Ltd
Phoenix Estate, Caerphilly Road, Cardiff CF4 4XG

Sinclair Pharmaceuticals Ltd
Borough Road, Godalming, Surrey GU7 2AB

Smith & Nephew Pharmaceuticals Ltd
PO Box 7, Bessemer Road, Welwyn Garden City, Herts AL7 1HF

Smith Kline & French Laboratories Ltd
Welwyn Garden City, Herts AL7 1EY

Spodefell Ltd
4 Inverness Mews, London W2 3JQ

E. R. Squibb & Sons Ltd
Squibb House, 141–149 Staines Road, Hounslow TW3 3JB

Stafford-Miller Ltd
Stafford-Miller House, The Common, Hatfield, Herts AL10 0NZ

Standard Laboratories Ltd
Windmill Road, Sunbury on Thames, Middlesex TW16 7DT

STD Pharmaceutical Products Ltd
6–7 Broad Street, Hereford HR4 9AE

Sterling Health Products
Sterling-Winthrop House, Surbiton, Surrey KT6 4PH

Sterling Research Laboratories
St Mark's Hill, Surbiton, Surrey KT6 4PH

Stiefel Laboratories (UK) Ltd
10 Wellcroft Road, Slough, Berks SL1 4AQ

Stuart Pharmaceuticals Ltd
Carr House, Carrs Road, Cheadle, Cheshire SK8 2EG

Syntex Pharmaceuticals Ltd
St Ives House, St Ives Road, Maidenhead, Berks SL6 1RD

Tillotts Laboratories
Unit 24, Henlow Trading Estate, Henlow, Beds SG16 6DS

Tosara Products Ltd
59 Crosby Road North, Liverpool L22 4QD

Travenol Laboratories Ltd
Caxton Way, Thetford, Norfolk IP24 3SE

Typharm Ltd
45 East Street, Blandford Forum, Dorset DT11 7DX

Unigreg Ltd
15–17 Worple Road, Wimbledon, London SW19 4JS

Unimed Pharmaceuticals Ltd
24 Steynton Avenue, Bexley, Kent DA5 3HP

Upjohn Ltd
Fleming Way, Crawley, West Sussex RH10 2NJ

Vitabiotics Ltd
122 Mount Pleasant, Alperton, Wembley, Middlesex HA0 1UG

Wade Pharmaceuticals Ltd
Stepfield, Wiltham, Essex CM8 3AG

Wallace Ltd
1a Frognal, London NW3 6AN

Wander Pharmaceuticals
98 The Centre, Feltham, Middlesex TW13 4EP

William R. Warner & Co. Ltd
Usk Road, Pontypool, Gwent NP4 0YH

WB Pharmaceuticals Ltd
PO Box 23, Bracknell, Berks RG12 4YS

Weddel Pharmaceuticals Ltd
Weddel House, 14 West Smithfield, London EC1A 9HY

Welbeck Medical Distributors Ltd
79 Wimpole Street, London W1M 7DD

Welfare Foods Ltd
63 London Road South, Poynton, Stockport, Cheshire SK12 1LA

Wellcome Medical Division
The Wellcome Foundation Ltd, Crewe Hall, Crewe, Cheshire CW1 1UB

Westminster Laboratories Ltd
Reckitt & Colman, Pharmaceutical Division, Dansom Lane, Hull HU8 7DS

Whatman Biochemicals
Springfield Mill, Maidstone, Kent ME14 2LE

Winthrop Laboratories
Sterling-Winthrop House, Surbiton, Surrey KT6 4PH

G. O. Woodward & Co. Ltd
Larkhall Laboratories, 225 Putney Bridge Road, London SW15 2PY

Wyeth Laboratories
Huntercombe Lane South, Taplow, Maidenhead, Berks SL6 0PH

Zyma (UK) Ltd
Hurdsfield Industrial Estate, Macclesfield, Cheshire SK10 2LY

□ *Operative Procedures*

Operative procedures: A to Z directory

Like all medical specialists surgeons have their own language and although one or two of the terms used to describe operations are well known there is little doubt that many patients find the language incomprehensible. On the following pages I have listed and explained some of the words used to describe the operations and techniques most commonly performed. Many of the words used have a different meaning when employed in a surgical context from the meaning they have when used in ordinary conversation. This list is not, of course, comprehensive, but many of the words which do not appear here can be translated if the basic language of surgery is understood.

For example, any word which ends in '-ectomy' suggests that a removal operation is implied (as in 'tonsillectomy') while the ending '-otomy' suggests that an incision will be made in some specific organ (as in 'laparotomy'). The ending '-plasty' suggests that a remoulding or plastic surgery operation is contemplated (as in 'mammaplasty') while the ending '-orrhaphy' means that a repair is intended (as in 'herniorrhaphy'). The other common ending is '-ostomy' and that means that the surgeon intends to form an artificial opening (as in 'colostomy').

achillorrhaphy Suturing of the Achilles tendon.

adenectomy Excision of a gland.

adenoidectomy Excision of the adenoids (usually refers to the removal of a mass of gland tissue in the region of a child's throat).

adipectomy Excision of adipose (fatty) tissue.

adrenalectomy Removal of an adrenal gland.

alveolotomy Making an incision in the alveolar process (near a tooth socket).

amniotomy Deliberately rupturing the foetal membranes, usually done to induce labour.

amputation Removal of a limb or any other bodily appendage.

anastomosis A surgical joining together of two tubular organs – for example a joining of two pieces of bowel.

aneurysmectomy Excision of an aneurysm (a dilated piece of artery).

angiectomy Excision of a part of a blood vessel.

annuloplasty A repair of any ring-shaped organ or area.

antrectomy Excision of a chamber or cavity – usually in bone.

aortotomy Cutting open the aorta.

apicectomy Resection of a tooth root, or indeed of any other apical structure.

aponeurectomy Excision of a sheet of tendon around a muscle.

apophysectomy Removal of a specific piece of bone.

appendectomy Removal of the appendix.

appendicectomy Removal of the appendix

apronectomy Plastic surgery operation to remove abdominal fat.

arterioplasty Repair of an artery.

arthrectomy Excision of a joint.

arthrodesis Surgical fixing of a joint so that there is no more movement.

aspiration The withdrawal of fluid.

autopsy Examination of a dead body.

avulsion Taking away a piece of tissue, usually by a tearing movement.

biopsy Taking a tissue sample for examination.

blepharectomy Excision of an eyelid.

block Usually means obstructing the passage of nervous impulses.

breech Literally means the buttock; a term used by obstetricians to refer to a baby appearing buttocks first instead of the more usual head first.

bronchoscopy Examination of the main tubes in the lungs with a special instrument.

bunionectomy Removal of a bunion.

burrholes Holes made in the skull.

bypass Operation which involves the use of an alternative route within the body (for example, a coronary bypass involves the building of an alternative route for blood supplying the heart).

Caesarian section *see* Cesarian section.

capsulectomy Excision of a capsule which is usually the enclosing membranous structure.

cardiomyotomy Operation to open the heart muscle.

castration Removal of the gonads to make the individual concerned incapable of reproducing (in men this operation is known as orchidectomy, in women it is oophorectomy).

cauterization Use of a hot instrument or caustic substance to destroy tissue.

cephalotomy The same as a craniotomy, which is a cutting open of the skull and usually refers to an operation performed on the foetus during a very difficult labour.

Cesarian section (or Caesarian section) Delivery of a baby through an incision made in the abdomen and uterus (or womb). Done if delivery is delayed or difficult for any reason.

chemosurgery Surgery which uses chemicals.

cholangiostomy Cutting open a bile duct.

cholecystectomy Cutting out the gall bladder.

chondrectomy Excision of a cartilage.

circumcision Excision of the foreskin in a male and clitoridotomy in a female.

clipping Use of clips (usually made of metal) to seal an opening or broken blood vessel.

clitoridectomy Excision of the clitoris.

clitoridotomy Incision or making a cut in the clitoris.

closure Sealing an opening. After an operation the incision has to be 'closed'.

colectomy Excision of the colon.

colorrhaphy Suture of the colon.

colostomy Bringing an end of the cut colon onto the abdominal surface and making a fistula out of it. The colostomy effectively acts as an artificial anus. Special sealed bags are used to collect the excreta.

colpectomy Removal of the vagina.

colporrhaphy Suture of the vagina.

cosmetic surgery Any operation done to improve the appearance of the patient.

craniectomy Cutting out part of the skull.

craniotomy Cutting open the skull.

cricoidectomy Cutting out the cricoid cartilage.

cryptorchidopexy Bringing an undescended testicle down into the scrotum and fixing it there.

curettage Cleaning of a body surface with a spoon-shaped instrument.

cystectomy Removal of a cyst. Or may mean removal of the urinary bladder.

D and C Dilatation and curettage: the cervix is dilated, a spoon-shaped instrument is inserted into the womb and the surface inside subjected to curettage.

debridement Removal of all foreign and contaminated material and tissue.

decompression Removal of pressure. For example, if there is excessive pressure inside the skull, a decompression operation may be performed by opening the skull.

defibrillation If a heart is beating irregularly-irregularly (in other words, if it is irregular but there is no pattern to the irregularity) it is said to be

fibrillating. A shock of some kind may sometimes stimulate the heart to begin beating normally again.

denervation Interruption or removal of a nerve supply to an organ or piece of tissue.

dialysis In scientific terms dialysis simply means the unidirectional movement of soluble molecules through a special type of membrane. In normal circumstances the human kidneys, for example, perform a function of this type. When the kidneys are not working properly 'artificial dialysis' may be required.

diathermy When high-frequency electric currents are passed through human tissues there is resistance and heat is produced. Surgeons use diathermy equipment to enable them to cut tissues without producing excessive bleeding.

dilation (or dilatation) Any process of expanding or enlarging.

disarticulation Amputation of a limb or part of a limb at a joint.

dissection In surgery, this means a separation of tissues.

diverticulectomy Excision of a diverticulum or blind pouch.

drainage Withdrawing fluids or other discharges from the body.

duodenectomy Excision of the duodenum.

embolectomy Removal of an embolus or mass in a blood vessel. May be a blood clot.

endarterectomy Clearing out of a partially blocked artery to help improve the blood flow.

enterocolostomy Anastomosis (or joining) of the small intestines to the colon.

enucleation Removal of any organ, tumour or indeed anything else in such a way that it comes out of the body quite whole.

epididymectomy Excision of the epididymis.

episiotomy Incision of the perineum. Small operation frequently done to facilitate childbirth.

evacuation Removal of material from the body through a natural passageway.

evisceration Removal of the inner parts of the body.

evulsion The forcible tearing away of a part of the body.

excision A cutting out.

exploration An investigative operation.

exposure An operation designed to make a previously hidden part of the body more accessible.

extraction Pulling out or removing some item (not necessarily a tooth).

fasciectomy Removal of a fascia or sheet of tissue around a muscle.

fenestration Perforating, or making a hole in something.

fusion Joining together.

gastrectomy Removal of the stomach (either partial or total).

graft To replace damaged or injured tissue with healthy tissue taken from another part of the same body or from another body.

hemorrhoidectomy (or haemorrhoidectomy) Excision of piles.

hepatectomy Excision of the liver.

herniorrhaphy Repair of a hernia.

hymenectomy Excision of the hymen (the membrane within the vagina of a female virgin).

hypophysectomy Removal of a small specific part of the brain (the hypophysis).

hysterectomy Excision of the uterus or womb.

hysterotomy Opening of the uterus or womb (sometimes done to facilitate the removal of a foetus, in which case it may be known as a Cesarian section or an abortion, depending on the state of the foetus).

ileectomy Excision of the ileum (part of the small intestine).

ileocolostomy An anastomosis (joining) of the ileum to the colon.

ileostomy An operation to bring the cut end of the ileum directly onto the abdominal surface (making an artificial anus which is then fitted with a special seal over which plastic collecting bags can be fixed).

implant To put a solid substance of any kind into the body for any reason (a metal hipjoint is an implant as is any medication source placed within the body to dissolve slowly).

incision Cut or opening.

induction Causing something to occur (e.g. an abortion).

intubation Putting a tube into a suitable bodily orifice. Generally speaking intubation is used to describe the putting of a tube into the larynx prior to the provision of a general anaesthetic.

intussusception reduction An intussusception occurs when one part of the intestine telescopes into another. Pulling the intussuscepted bowel back into place is called reducing it.

iridectomy Excision of the iris within the eye.

jejunectomy Excision of the jejunum (the part of the small intestine which runs between the duodenum and the ileum).

laminectomy Excision of part of a vertebral bone.

laparotomy Opening the abdomen. Usually done as an investigative operation.

laryngectomy Removal of the larynx.

lavage A washing out.

leucotomy (or leukotomy) Cutting of the white matter at the front of the brain in order to interrupt the passage of messages within the brain and so affect thought processes.

ligation A tying off, or application of a ligature made of thread or wire.

lipectomy Removal of fatty tissue.

lithotomy Cutting open an organ to remove a stone. Usually refers to the bladder.

lobectomy Removal of a lobe (e.g. of a lung, the liver etc.).

lumpectomy Removal of a lump of any kind anywhere in the body.

lymphadenectomy Removal of lymph gland tissue.

mammoplasty Redesign of breast shape and size. May be a reduction operation (designed to make a large breast smaller) or an augmentation operation (designed to make a small breast larger).

mastectomy Removal of breast tissue. A radical mastectomy involves the removal of surrounding tissues as well.

mastoidectomy Removal of the mastoid bone.

meniscectomy Removal of the semi-lunar cartilage of the knee joint.

myectomy Excision of muscle.

myotomy Cutting open a muscle.

nephrectomy Removal of a kidney.

obliteration A complete removal of tissue.

oophorectomy Removal of one or both ovaries.

orchidectomy Removal of one or both testes.

ostectomy Removal of bone.

osteotomy Incision of a bone.

otoplasty Plastic repair of the ear.

pancreatectomy Removal of the pancreas gland.

panhysterectomy Complete removal of the womb and cervix.

papillectomy Removal of a papilla.

parathyroidectomy Removal of the parathyroid gland.

phlebotomy Incision or opening of a vein.

pneumonectomy Removal of lung tissue.

polypectomy Removal of a polyp.

prostatectomy Removal of all or part of the prostate gland.

pyloroplasty Repair or redesign of the pylorus which marks the boundary between the stomach and the duodenum.

reduction The restoration of the normal relationship between parts of the body. Fractures and hernias, for example, are said to be reduced when repaired.

resection The surgical removal of a piece of tissue — usually quite a large part of the organ concerned.

revascularization The repair or restoration of the blood supply to a part of the body.

rhinoplasty Plastic surgery repair of the nose.

rhytidectomy Plastic removal of wrinkles (usually on the face and around the eyes).

salpingo-oophorectomy Excision of fallopian tube and ovary (can be bilateral or unilateral).

screening Any procedure designed to identify a dangerous disorder at an early stage.

section A cutting (as in a Cesarian section).

shunt A diversion (usually refers to a bypass or anastomosis, designed to deliver blood around some obstacle).

sinusotomy Incision of a sinus.

sphincterotomy Cutting of a sphincter.

splenectomy Removal of the spleen.

stapedectomy Removal of the stapes bone from the ear.

sterilization Operation done to provide a permanent contraceptive effect.

suspension An operation designed to provide a support or sling for a part of the body.

suture A repair using silk, catgut, nylon, cotton thread or wire stitches.

sympathectomy Cutting of a sympathetic nerve.

synovectomy Removal of a synovial membrane.

syringing Clearing a body cavity with fluids deliberately introduced with the aid of an instrument. Ears filled with wax are commonly syringed.

tap An operation in which fluid is withdrawn from a part of the body.

tenotomy Cutting of a tendon.

termination Abortion.

thrombectomy Removal of a clot.

thyroidectomy Removal of the thyroid gland.

tonsillectomy Removal of the tonsils.

tracheostomy Making a hole in the trachea or windpipe. Usually done as an emergency when some obstruction prevents normal breathing.

traction Drawing or pulling.

transfusion Introducing blood or some other fluid into the body.

transplantation Grafting of tissues from another part of the body or another body altogether.

ureterotomy Cutting open a ureter (the duct from the kidney to the bladder).

vaginoplasty Plastic repair of the vagina.

vagotomy Cutting of the vagus nerve (often done in conjunction with operations on the stomach).

valvotomy Cutting of a valve, particularly a valve of the heart.

vasectomy Excision of the vas deferens. Used as a method of sterilization in the male.

venesection Opening a vein to withdraw blood for any reason.

venipuncture The surgical opening of a vein with a needle or small instrument.

ventrosuspension Fixing a retroverted uterus so that it is suspended from the abdominal wall.

version To turn around (for example, a foetus within the womb).

vulvectomy The removal of the vulva.

□ *Other Forms of Treatment*

Other forms of treatment: A to Z directory

Most of the treatments advocated by medical practitioners involve either drugs or surgery. There are, however, many other forms of treatment which play an important part in medical care. In the following list I have described in brief detail some of the other remedies available.

abreaction
With the aid of some drugs patients may be encouraged to recall and even relive forgotten episodes which may have produced psychic scars. This type of treatment is called abreaction.

electroconvulsive therapy (ECT)
This extremely controversial form of treatment involves the use of large amounts of electricity on the human brain. The advocates argue that ECT has helped many individuals. The opponents argue that it is barbaric and dangerous. There is no completely conclusive evidence for or against electroconvulsive therapy.

occupational therapy
Occupational therapists are not solely concerned with ensuring that their patients have something to do; they also play an important part in preparing convalescent patients for future employment. Occupational therapy is, therefore, commonly prescribed by physicians looking after an individual who has been ill for some time with either a chronic or a recurring problem (*see* p. 130).

physiotherapy
Patients with muscular weaknesses and bony disorders of any kind are often referred to the local physiotherapy department. Special exercises and treatments are available there to help relieve muscle and joint pain and to help improve the rate at which weakened muscles regain strength.

psychotherapy
In psychotherapy the doctor-patient relationship is of paramount importance. The doctor or psychotherapist will spend many months or even years talking to the patient and providing support and understanding. Because this form of treatment usually involves a one-to-one relationship and may last for a considerable amount of time it is not widely available within the health service.

radiotherapy

Marie and Pierre Curie were the first to discover the value of radiation therapy and their early work on radium earned them international recognition. Today, radiotherapy is regarded as an important form of treatment for many conditions. It is one of the most important weapons available to doctors who specialize in the treatment of cancer. Radium, incidentally, is a rare substance emitting several different rays which have varying penetration power. It is those rays which are used in the treatment of diseased tissues.

transfusion

The fluids circulating in the body have a number of important jobs to do. When the total quantity of fluid in the body drops (as it may after a heavy bleed, for example) the survival of the body may be threatened. Lost fluid may be replaced by blood or by other specially prepared and formulated fluids. Transfusion is simply the introduction into the body circulation of any fluid.

Home Care

Learning how to care at home

For several reasons the enthusiasm and ability of individuals to deal effectively with simple health care problems at home has changed considerably in recent years.

One reason is undoubtedly the partial breakdown in the strength of the traditional family unit. For example, it used to be possible for a young mother with a fractious child or complaining husband to seek basic advice from her own mother or an aunt. With the building of so many new housing estates, the increased mobility of young families and the reduced importance of family ties it is relatively rare for a young woman today to seek advice from such a source. Alone and without experience she inevitably turns to the professionals. Her eagerness to seek professional advice will have undoubtedly been greatly enhanced by the medical profession's too well publicized enthusiasm for its own forms of treatment. The power of the many new available drugs, the healing capacity of the surgical knife and the mystical qualities of the many electrical devices currently used by doctors in all specialities will have contributed to her excess of faith and enthusiasm.

The truth, however, is rather different. The fact is that the majority of simple, uncomplicated disorders are best treated at home. Old-fashioned symptomatic remedies are safer than more modern solutions and are often just as effective. And there are additional benefits to be gained by learning the rudimentary facts about home health care.

First, of course, it is more convenient and less expensive to deal with simple problems at home. If you need to visit a doctor and obtain a prescription for an attack of catarrh the cost in terms of time and money can be high. If you know how to deal

303

with the problem yourself the cost can be almost negligible. And, of course, there is no need to wait for an appointment or for the doctor to visit. The individual or family who can limit the number of times that professional care is sought will benefit in a number of important ways. Inevitably, for example, the doctor who has not been troubled for an apparently unending series of minor ailments will be more likely to deal sympathetically and effectively with a real problem when and if it arises. Doctors try not to become blasé when their patients cry wolf but it is difficult to maintain concentration and interest if the patient asking for help is recognized as one who frequently attends with truly trivial problems. One important additional benefit which may accrue if patients learn how best to use their doctors will undoubtedly be an increase in the time available for dealing with serious problems. The family doctor who sees thirty people with coughs and colds in a single surgery has that much less time to spend on an individual who comes in with a genuinely threatening complaint.

But the real advantage which is associated with sensible self care is far more important than the ones I have mentioned so far. If you attend a screening clinic once a year then you are 'safe' for a week or so afterwards. You stand a better chance of keeping out of trouble if you learn to screen yourself all the time. Permanent self-screening, or learning to listen to your body so that you can tell without delay when it gives you warning that something is wrong, is the most important facet of home health care.

There are now a great many bits and pieces of equipment on sale to those who want to look after their own health and identify dangers at an early stage. It is possible to buy cancer-testing kits, sphygmomanometers for home use, do-it-yourself urine-testing kits and even a bra which is said to enable the wearer to tell if she is developing breast cancer. But I do not believe that any of these gadgets are as necessary or as effective as the acquisition of a little knowledge about exactly what to look for and which symptoms to take seriously. After all, the most important question which any individual threatened by ill health has to answer is not 'What needs to be done?' but 'Do I need professional help?'. Where there is nothing more threatening than inconvenient symptoms to be dealt with the good home nurse can provide the solution just as easily as the skilled physician. Where there are dangerous symptoms to be investigated the advice of a physician is indispensable.

This book is not intended to provide a guide to home health care but I have included here short notes on simple home screening and on preparing and using a home medicine cabinet. Two other books of mine, *Aspirin or Ambulance?* (published in paperback by Jill Norman) and *The Home Pharmacy* (published in paperback by Pan Books), are intended to provide a more comprehensive outline to the provision of good home health care. The first of these two books, *Aspirin or Ambulance?*, is designed to help readers answer for themselves the simple question: 'Do we need a doctor?', while the second book, *The Home Pharmacy*, is intended to provide answers for the family or individual looking for symptomatic relief and wanting to know which products to choose for which symptoms.

I mention my own books because if I did not have faith in them I would not have allowed them to be published but there are, of course, many hundreds of other volumes available for those who wish to improve their ability to care for minor problems at home. In particular there is a large number of books on sale dealing with specific problems in depth and providing details and explanations about the pathology of specific disorders and about the forms of treatment available. I heartily recommend anyone suffering from a chronic disorder to get in touch with the association providing care and assistance for sufferers from that disorder (see pp. 174–84). Most such organizations publish recommended book lists.

Finally, I think it worthwhile mentioning that two organizations, the British Medical Association and the Health Education Council, publish a vast number of booklets and leaflets on specific medical topics. The Health Education Council publishes many free leaflets on a wide range of subjects and a copy of their

Home screening:
some major warning signs

You should see a doctor without delay if:

1 You have any unexplained pain which recurs or which is present for more than five days (obviously, severe pains need to be investigated without delay)

2 You have any unexplained bleeding – from anywhere

3 You need to take any home medicine regularly or for five days or more

4 You notice any persistent change in your body (e.g. a loss or gain in weight, a paralysis of any kind, or the development of any lump or swelling)

5 Any existing lump, wart or other skin blemish changes size or colour or bleeds

6 You notice new symptoms when you have already received medical treatment

7 There are mental symptoms present such as confusion, paranoia, disorientation or severe depression

up-to-date publications list can be obtained from their offices at 78 New Oxford Street, London WC1A 1AH. The British Medical Association publishes a wide range of inexpensive 'Family Doctor' booklets dealing with pregnancy and childbirth, childcare management, sex education, dieting, general health and psychological problems. These booklets are available from chemists or from Family Doctor Publications, BMA House, Tavistock Square, London WC1H 9JP. The 'Family Doctor' list of publications includes specific volumes on diabetes, epilepsy, rheumatism, blood pressure, ulcers, headaches, heart attacks and the menopause.

The Home Medicine Chest

Every home should have a medicine cabinet which is properly stocked. Ideally, of course, a medicine cabinet should have a lock so that the medicines inside it can be locked out of the reach of small children. Although medicine cabinets are traditionally kept in the bathroom this really is not the best place for drugs since the variations in temperature which occur may accelerate the rate at which drugs deteriorate. Any room which has a more or less constant temperature is suitable.

Before stocking up with suitable home remedies it is a good idea to clear out all the half-empty, improperly labelled bottles which will probably have accumulated over the years. Anything that is not clearly labelled should be thrown away and anything more than six, or at the most twelve, months old should also be discarded. Tablets and medicines can be flushed down the lavatory.

It does not cost much to stock up a basic home medicine cabinet and the total cost can be kept down by buying non-branded products.

1 A pain reliever such as soluble aspirin or paracetamol tablets. The advantage of paracetamol is that you can buy it in liquid form as well as in tablets. The doses for children

307

and adults should be on the bottles. Incidentally, a hot-water bottle is also an excellent pain reliever. Wrapped in a pillow case or thin towel it can be held against a painful ear, abdomen or joint and will often provide a great deal of relief.

2 An indigestion remedy. Again you do not need to buy a branded product. There are many suitable preparations on the market but ordinary aluminium hydroxide mixture or tablets will probably be suitable for most people's occasional indigestion upsets.

3 A laxative. Bran is one of the simplest and most natural types of laxative and although some individuals may complain that their bowels are already so addicted to chemical laxatives that bran will not work I do recommend that whenever possible the more powerful products are avoided.

4 An anti-diarrhoeal medicine. Something simple, such as kaolin mixture, is probably as good as anything else you can buy.

5 An inhalant. Catarrh and sinus troubles are extremely common in Britain and the best way to deal with them is to inhale the steam rising from a bowl of hot (not boiling) water. If a menthol crystal is added to the water the effect will be even more dramatic.

6 A bottle of calamine lotion to help with itchy spots and rashes.

I suggest that only small quantities of these medicines be bought, since anyone who is really likely to use a Monster 500 tablet package of aspirins really needs to see a doctor. In addition to these medicines the cabinet can also be stocked with whatever bandages, instruments and fabric plasters you feel capable of using.

My book, *The Home Pharmacy* (published by Pan Books), contains a comprehensive account of the over-the-counter or non-prescription medication available in Britain.

Health Insurance

☐ *Statutory Schemes*

☐ *Private Schemes*

☐ *Statutory Schemes*

Rights and regulations

The social security section of the Department of Health and Social Security hands out millions of pounds every year. It is an undoubted fact that although much of that money is taken by people who do not need it and are not entitled to it, many thousands of people fail to claim money which they do need and to which they are entitled. The rules and regulations governing the distribution of social security benefits are complex and ever-changing, and the sums of money involved also change quite frequently. This section is intended not to provide a comprehensive account of the enormous variety of rights and regulations governing the distribution of benefits but to serve as a brief introductory guide through the complex maze devised by the DHSS.

To begin with it is important to understand that social security benefits fall into two main categories: contributory benefits and non-contributory benefits. As the name suggests the benefits in the first category are paid to those individuals (or their relatives) who have paid specific sums of money to the government over a period of time as national insurance stamps, pension contributions and so on. Before contributory benefits can be paid out the officers of the social security office will want to be satisfied that claimants have paid the necessary number of contributions and that their current circumstances (age, state of health etc.) entitle them to make a claim. Non-contributory benefits, on the other hand, are paid to anyone who can make a justifiable claim and they are not dependent on any contributions having been made. Some non-contributory benefits, however, are only paid after a means test has been applied.

The DHSS publishes an enormous range of leaflets designed to explain the rules and regulations in precise detail. I suggest that you ask your local office for the appropriate leaflets if you are considering a claim. If the leaflets you want are not forthcoming, do not be discouraged. When my wife went to a social security office to pick up a range of leaflets for me she was told by a counter clerk that people are not supposed to have leaflets in any quantity. Since many leaflets cross-refer this could be a problem. So tell a reluctant clerk to read leaflet NI146 carefully Rule-conscious clerks should then give you as many leaflets as you are likely to want.

One of the most important leaflets is called 'Which benefit?' and subtitled '60 ways to get cash help'. This leaflet is officially. known as FB2. If you have difficulty in obtaining a copy from the local social security office then you can obtain a copy by writing to DHSS Leaflets Unit, PO Box 21, Stanmore, Middlesex HA7 1AY, quoting the reference number FB2.

Contributory benefits

Generally speaking everyone between the age of sixteen and retirement age has to pay national insurance contributions while working. Employers also have to pay contributions for their employees. A small part of the money paid in this way helps finance the National Health Service. But most of the money helps pay for the benefits paid out to people making claims. The people paying contributions today are providing the money for the people making claims today.

Class 1 contributions are paid by people working for employers. The rate of contribution varies according to the level of earning. Contributors in this class are entitled to all contributory benefits.

Class 2 contributions are paid by the self-employed, who are also liable to pay Class 4 contributions on any profits they make. These Class 4 contributions are paid directly to the Inland Revenue and do not have any effect on claims which may be made. Class 2 contributors are entitled to all contributory benefits except unemployment benefit.

Class 3 contributions are paid by people who for some reason have not made enough Class 1 or Class 2 contributions and who want to be able to make claims in the future. Class 3 contributors are entitled to all contributory benefits except unemployment benefit, sickness benefit, invalidity benefit and maternity allowance.

Each contributor has a national insurance number which he or she keeps for life. That number is used to help keep a record of contributions made. Individuals who are unemployed, sick or in training may be credited with contributions instead of having to pay them.

The main types of contributory benefit are described below.

Unemployment benefit

This is payable only to Class 1 contributors, and only when a contributor has been employed for a fixed period and has registered as fit and capable of work at the appropriate office. Unemployment benefit is payable for up to 312 days but cannot be claimed again without a further period of employment. Contributors who voluntarily leave employment may not be entitled to benefit. Prior to January 1982 an earnings related supplement was paid.

People who lose their jobs and who have worked for the same employer for at least two years may be entitled to redundancy payments and tax rebates.

Sickness benefit

Sickness benefit is paid to Class 1 and Class 2 contributors. It is paid for 28 weeks only and is then replaced by invalidity benefit. A certificate entitling an individual to claim sickness benefit can be obtained from a GP or, in the case of a hospital in-patient, from a representative of the hospital.

Invalidity benefit and allowance

When sickness benefit stops, after 28 weeks of illness, contributors can claim invalidity pensions. People who become chronically ill before reaching the age of sixty (for men) or fifty-five (for women) can also claim an invalidity allowance. The size of the invalidity allowance varies according to the age at which incapacity began.

Maternity benefit

Maternity benefit is made up of a maternity grant and a maternity allowance. The former is paid to all pregnant women who have themselves paid national insurance contributions or whose husbands have done so. Class 1, 2 and 3 contributors are eligible for the maternity grant. The money is usually handed over on production of a certificate of expected confinement signed by a midwife or GP only when the pregnancy has reached 26 weeks.

Maternity benefit also includes a maternity allowance which is payable to women who have paid Class 1 or 2 contributions. It can be claimed when the pregnancy has reached 26 weeks, and is paid for up to 18 weeks as long as the woman is not still working.

In addition, a woman who stops work to have a baby and has worked for the same employer for two years or more may be able to claim paid maternity leave from her employer.

Finally, all expectant mothers are entitled to free milk and vitamins, and free dental treatment and prescriptions.

Child's special allowance

A divorced woman with a child can claim this allowance if her ex-husband dies and he has been paying child maintenance and contributions of Class 1, 2 or 3. The allowance is not paid to a woman who remarries.

Widow's benefit

Widow's benefit is divided into three parts: widow's pension, widow's allowance and widowed mother's allowance.

All these benefits are paid to all women whose late husbands have paid contributions of any class.

The widow's allowance is paid to women who are under the age of sixty on the death of their husbands (or over sixty if their husbands were still working). They receive a weekly payment for the first 26 weeks of widowhood. The payment is increased if there are children.

When the 26 weeks of widow's allowance are finished, the widow with one or more dependent children will receive the widowed mother's allowance, while the widow without any dependent children may be able to claim a widow's pension under certain circumstances. The rules surrounding the widow's pension are rather complicated, but no widow under the age of forty is entitled to payment.

Retirement pension

A man of sixty-five and a woman of sixty can, on retiring from full-time employment, obtain a pension if sufficient contributions have been made. Individuals can under some circumstances claim non-contributory pensions if they are over eighty years of age.

The rules governing the payment of pensions and graduated pensions are rather complex but a claim form is usually sent to all eligible contributors automatically and there are a number of suitable leaflets available which explain the rules in detail.

Death grant

If a Class 1, 2 or 3 contributor, or his or her spouse or child, dies, a death grant may be payable to the next of kin or person paying the funeral expenses. The rate of the grant varies according to the age of the deceased.

Non-contributory benefits

To obtain non-contributory benefits individuals must only show that they meet certain conditions. Some benefits are only paid after means tests have been applied.

Here are some of the non-contributory benefits which can be claimed.

Injury benefit and disablement benefit

Employees who are injured at work or who contract diseases as a result of their employment may be entitled to industrial injuries benefit. The injury or disease must have arisen out of and in the course of employment and it must usually have happened in Great Britain. Any accidents must be reported and any disease suspected of being related to working hazards has to be assessed by a doctor other than the patient's own GP.

There are two types of benefit paid – injury benefit (paid for 26 weeks only) and disablement benefit (which is not limited and which can be paid even when an employee is still able to work). According to the latest leaflet published by the DHSS there are fifty-one diseases prescribed under the industrial injuries scheme. The leaflet listing these diseases is known as NI2. The leaflet which describes injury benefit for accidents at work is NI5.

Child benefit

Families with one or more children can claim a cash payment each week. The payment is not subject to any earnings rule.

Family income supplement

Anyone bringing up children on low earnings from full-time work can claim family income supplement. The amount of money paid depends on the amount of money being earned and on the number of children. In addition to being paid cash,

315

claimants may be entitled to free school meals, free milk and vitamins, free NHS dental treatment, free spectacles and free prescriptions.

Supplementary benefit

Individuals of 16 or over who are not working full time and who do not have enough money to live on can claim supplementary benefit. The benefit is not paid if the individual has savings of more than a certain amount. Claimants over pension age may be entitled to claim a supplementary pension. Many people are entitled to supplementary benefits but do not claim them.

Attendance allowance

Severely disabled individuals who need frequent attention or constant supervision can claim a home attendance allowance. The mentally as well as the physically ill are entitled to this allowance as are children over the age of two. Claimants must have been ill for six months or more.

Invalid care allowance

Men and single women of working age who cannot go out to work because they have to stay at home to look after someone receiving an attendance allowance may be entitled to claim an invalid care allowance.

Mobility allowance

Individuals between the ages of five and sixty-five who are physically disabled and unable to walk may be entitled to a mobility allowance.

Non-contributory invalidity pension

People of working age who have not paid enough national insurance contributions to get invalidity benefit, but who have been unable to work for at least six months may be entitled to claim the NCIP. Married women who are unable to do normal housework may also be able to claim a housewife's non-contributory invalidity pension.

Guardian's allowance

A person who takes an orphan child into the family and who is entitled to child benefit for that child may also be entitled to claim a guardian's allowance.

Criminal injuries compensation

People injured as a result of a violent crime, and dependants of those killed as a result of a violent crime, may be entitled to compensation. An application form and leaflet can be obtained from the Criminal Injuries Compensation Board, 10–12 Russell Square, London WC1B 5EN. Claims must be made within three years of the date of injury.

There are, in addition, other ways in which people can claim money. People who find it difficult to pay their full rent or rates may be entitled to rent or rate rebates. Individuals injured while serving with the armed forces may be entitled to special payments.

The most important source of information about all these types of payment is the leaflet 'Which Benefit?' which I have already described (see p. 311).

☐ *Private Schemes*

The variety of schemes available

With the demand for private medical care on the increase, it is hardly surprising that there has in recent years been a comparable rise in the demand for private health care insurance. In all countries where medical care is provided on a fee basis (rather than through a state-run organization) there are insurance companies offering to provide individuals with some way of insuring their own health and minimizing the financial damage which might be incurred as a result of an accident or illness.

The best established and best known type of insurance scheme is the sort that simply offers to pay medical costs for any unexpected episode of illness in return for a regular payment. The customers of such organizations are simply insuring their own health in much the same way as they might insure their home or motor cars.

In recent years, the demand for this type of health care insurance has grown dramatically, and today well over half of all the individuals using private medical care facilities are covered by one or other of the insurance companies which exist.

The two most well-known companies, British United Provident Association (BUPA) and Private Patients Plan (PPP) have between them 98 per cent of the market in Britain and both offer group rates as well as individual terms. It is no longer only companies' buying cover for their executives that makes up most of the group insurance business for these two organizations; today there are many trade unions which have a negotiated cover for their members. The official Labour party policy opposing the growth of private medical care is clearly not adhered to in practice by many of the party's supporters. Policemen, engineers and electricians are just three of the groups of workers widely involved in buying private insurance.

At the moment, these organizations only pay medical costs for an illness or accident; none of the schemes will pay for private general practitioner care. One well-known scheme offering GP cover is the London based Medicover organization which for a fixed annual fee and a 'call out' fee will guarantee to provide any patient with a home visit at any time.

In recent years ordinary health insurance schemes have been joined by various other projects. One of the best advertised schemes is the one designed to pay subscribers a fixed amount of money for every day they need to spend in hospital.

The Sun Alliance Hospital Benefits Plan, for example, is designed to pay subscribers a fixed sum of money which varies according to the premium paid. The scheme includes optional and additional benefits so that if, for instance, a husband and wife both need to be admitted to hospital at the same time the benefit paid will be increased. Ambassador Life and Hospital Plan Insurance Services offer similar cover. Occasionally insurance cover of this kind can be linked to life insurance.

My personal view is that since many doctors and administrators are now trying to get patients out of hospital as quickly as possible (and to perform surgery on out-patients) ordinary sickness insurance, designed to provide payments for days lost from work rather than for days spent in hospital, might be a better buy. After all, it does not make much difference to the loss of income whether an individual is ill in hospital or ill at home; indeed when an individual is ill in hospital the housekeeping costs are likely to be lower. Local insurance brokers can usually offer a variety of ordinary sickness insurance schemes designed to provide general cover.

A more controversial type of insurance cover is that which provides parents-to-be with insurance against a child having any congenital handicap. The individual buying insurance will be paid if a child suffers from such disorders as spina bifida and cerebral palsy. Again, details of this type of insurance can be obtained from an ordinary insurance broker. As always, do read the small print of any such scheme carefully.

319

Finally, there are a number of schemes in existence which were founded many years ago to help support voluntary hospitals. When they were originally founded the Birmingham Hospital Saturday Fund, the Norfolk and Suffolk Hospitals Contributors Association and the Hospital Fund (Bradford and District) were designed to help pay for local hospitals. Today these, and other organizations which are in the British Hospitals Contributory Schemes Association, have a total of several million members who receive small sums of money when they are ill, get some NHS expenses paid, and are entitled to stay at convalescent homes run by their organizations. The address of the BHCSA is 30 Lancaster Gate, London W2 3LT, and a list of the twenty-eight affiliated contributory schemes can be obtained from the Honorary Secretary.

A final and special case of a private contributory scheme is the Manor House Hospital in London which is at least partly paid for by contributions made by industrial workers, and is in effect a private hospital run by and for workers in a variety of industries. It is reputed to have been given special permission to remain outside the NHS when the latter was founded in 1948.

Tips for choosing a private health insurance scheme

1 If you are planning on joining BUPA, PPP, or any other association offering health care insurance, it is wise to study all the available literature (and to read all the small print carefully) since the costs of cover and the services provided vary a good deal.

2 If you are offered membership of a group scheme with any association then you will probably pay less than if you join as an individual. Most individuals can easily arrange to be members of some group or other!

3 Look carefully at the cover you are being offered. The most expensive item in private medical care is the cost of the

hospital bed which will usually be several hundred pounds a week at the very least. So if you are only being offered a payment to the consultant you see, then the cover is of very limited value.

4 When buying health insurance it is important to be aware of the limitations of what you are buying. Unless you pay very high premiums you are unlikely to be covered for care in the most expensive private hospitals in London (where 'hotel' costs alone can exceed £1500 a week) and whatever you pay you may not be covered for cosmetic surgery or treatment from alternative care practitioners. Remember too that the availability of private care for emergency treatment is very limited, and that there are limitations on the treatment made available for the chronic sick or for patients who have existing disorders.

5 Before you buy health insurance make sure that there are private consultants and beds available in your area. In some parts of Britain there are few facilities for private practice, and you may in fact be choosing between treatment near home in an NHS hospital or treatment a long way away in a private ward. Local health service lists are also relevant, since in some parts of Britain the wait for a routine operation can be a matter of weeks while the wait for an identical operation in other parts of the country may be years.

Travelling at Home and Abroad

Anyone travelling abroad should have the necessary vaccinations (see p. 275) and should take with them a supply of any medication needed regularly. Health service general practitioners will usually provide patients with a supply for one month, but people intending to stay abroad for longer than that may need to obtain fresh supplies while abroad, and for this reason patients suffering from long-term medical problems should take with them a brief account of their medical history if they intend to stay abroad for more than a month (see also 'Medic Alert' etc. p. 337).

Most travel agents and insurance brokers will have details of health insurance schemes, many of which are run together with baggage and other general insurance. Britain has reciprocal health care arrangements with a number of countries (notably its fellow members of the European Economic Community) and details of these arrangements can be obtained by asking any local social security office for a copy of leaflet SA30. This leaflet not only includes details of all arrangements but also contains the application form for the certificate of entitlement (form E111) needed in countries in the EEC.

All travellers intending to journey outside Britain should obtain a copy of leaflet SA35 'Notice to travellers: health protection' published by the DHSS. This leaflet can be obtained free of charge from the International Relations Division, Room C511, Alexander Fleming House, Elephant and Castle, London SE1 6BY or through travel agents. The Health Education Council publishes a leaflet entitled 'Advice to travellers' (address p. 169).

British travellers who do not intend to journey outside their country are entitled to free medical care wherever they go, both from general practitioners and from the hospital service. When visiting a hospital as an emergency patient there should be no administrative problems; when visiting a general practitioner the patient will be asked to sign a form (FP19) as a temporary resident. After treatment, this form, on which the GP will record any notes he makes, will be sent to the patient's own home GP.

In 1981 the British government announced that visitors to Britain using the National Health Service would be expected to pay for treatment they received unless they had chosen to settle in Britain or had been resident for three years or more. Naturally visitors from countries having reciprocal health care arrangements with Britain (for example, countries within the European Economic Community) would not be charged.

When Someone Dies:
what has to be done

Deaths fall into two categories: the expected and the unexpected. When someone has been ill for some time and has been receiving medical care the procedure to be followed can be organized in advance. Either they will have been cared for in a hospital or nursing home, in which case the immediate arrangements can be left to the staff there, or they will have been cared for at home, in which case the GP who is in charge should be consulted about what may need to be done. In the case of an 'unexpected' death the coroner will usually have to be notified, and there may be a post mortem and sometimes an inquest.

Expected deaths

There are far more 'expected' than unexpected deaths, and of the total number of deaths each year in the United Kingdom only about one in ten is unexpected and reported to the coroner. The majority of those unexpected deaths are a result of heart disease and heart attacks. Only once in a lifetime does a doctor expect to deal with a genuinely 'unnatural' death.

The procedure to be followed when a death that has been expected occurs at home will usually have been explained beforehand. Some doctors expect as a matter of routine to be called at night if a patient who has been ill dies, while others do not. If the deceased is to be cremated, then the doctor must make an examination of the dead body, and indeed must arrange for a second, independent doctor to make an examination as well. Whatever plans exist for the deceased (burial or cremation, for example) a death certificate must be issued and taken to the local Registrar of Births, Marriages and Deaths. The doctor issuing the certificate will be able to provide the address of the local Registrar as will the funeral director given responsibility for making any necessary arrangements. Doctors cannot issue a death certificate unless they have looked after the patient during his or her last illness. If the patient has not been seen during the last fourteen days of his or her life then the doctor will probably refer the case to the coroner although this does not necessarily mean that any other action need be taken.

In hospital, many doctors like a post mortem to be performed routinely, even on patients who have died after a long, serious, identified illness. This is done as much to provide valuable clinical information as to ascertain the precise cause of death, and if relatives object strongly to the idea of a post mortem being carried out the investigation can, of course, be waived unless the doctor's application is supported by a coroner.

Unexpected deaths

In the case of what appears to be an unexpected death it is always best to regard the individual as being alive but ill rather than dead unless there really is no doubt at all. Many apparently moribund individuals have been brought back to life by the provision of immediate medical care. Telephoning for a general practitioner or an ambulance is obviously a priority, but anyone capable of carrying out simple life-saving procedures who finds an apparently dead body should act on the basis that the individual is unconscious but alive. (Obviously in some cases it will be immediately apparent that there is no point at all in attempting any resuscitation.) If there are obvious signs of violence then the police should be notified as well.

An unexpected death will usually have to be reported to the coroner whether or not there is any suspicion that the death was in any way unnatural. The coroner will then arrange for a pathologist to perform a post mortem. As a result of inquiries made on his behalf by the local police the coroner will then decide whether or not an inquest is necessary. If no inquest is necessary the coroner himself will issue the death certificate.

325

Other things to remember

In addition to making the practical arrangements for the funeral there may be other things for the bereaved to do.

First, you should find out as soon as possible whether the deceased had made any plans for the disposal of any part or the whole of his or her body. Individuals who want to leave their bodies to medical science can contact the professor of anatomy at a local medical school or HM Inspector of Anatomy at the Department of Health and Social Security in London. If these arrangements have been made then the local professor or the London Inspector must be notified as soon as possible after death. Similarly, if the deceased has bequeathed his or her eyes to the blind (usually through the Royal National Institute for the Blind) contact must be made with the receiving organization (see also p. 337 for information on organ donors). Second, it is important for all friends and relatives of the deceased to be aware of the pressure on the members of the immediate family. Depression after bereavement is natural but if there is any question of a need for medical aid then it should be sought sooner rather than later. It is also important for friends and relatives to assist the bereaved in any claims for death grants, widow's benefits and so on (see p. 314).

A comprehensive account of how to cope after death is contained in the book *What to do when someone dies* which is published by the Consumers' Association (the publishers of *Which?* magazine) and should be available in the reference sections of most public libraries; and the DHSS publishes a leaflet called 'What to do after a death' (D49) which can be obtained from your local social security office or from the DHSS Leaflets Unit, PO Box 21, Stanmore, Middlesex HA7 1AY.

General Information

A to Z directory of abbreviations commonly used in medicine

Abbreviations can often be dangerous. Doctors, nurses and others involved in the care of patients do not always mean the same thing when they use a particular abbreviation. For example, the letters IUD can mean both an intra-uterine device and an intra-uterine death. The list that follows is intended simply as an introductory guide to some of the most commonly used shorthand forms.

AA Alcoholics Anonymous

A7 Patient told to attend in seven days' time

ABPI Association of the British Pharmaceutical Industry

ACTH adrenocorticotropic hormone

AF atrial fibrillation

AHA Area Health Authority (now historical)

AI aortic incompetence OR artificial insemination

AMO Area Medical Officer (now historical)

AN ante-natal

ANS autonomic nervous system

AP antero-posterior

APH antepartum haemorrhage

AS aortic stenosis OR alimentary system

ASD atrial septal defect

A & W alive and well

BAOT British Association of Occupational Therapists

BBA born before arrival

BBD baby born dead

BDA British Dental Association

BE barium enema

BI bone injury

BID brought in dead

BM barium meal

BMA British Medical Association

BMR basal metabolic rate

BNF British National Formulary

BO bowels opened OR body odour

BP blood pressure OR British Pharmacopoeia

BPC British Pharmaceutical Codex

BUPA British United Provident Association

C centigrade OR certificate

C7 certificate given for 7 days

Ca	carcinoma		**DHSS**	Department of Health and Social Security
CCF	congestive cardiac failure		**DLE**	disseminated lupus erythematosus
CCHMS	Central Committee for Hospital Medical Services		**DMO**	divisional medical officer
CD	casualty department		**DN**	district nurse
CF	cardiac failure OR final certificate (sick note) given		**DNA**	did not attend
			DOA	dead on arrival
			DOB	date of birth
CHF	congestive heart failure		**DOM**	department of medicine
Cho/Vac	cholera vaccine		**DOS**	department of surgery
Circ	circumcision OR circulation		**DP/Vac**	diphtheria and pertussis vaccine
CNS	central nervous system		**DS**	disseminated sclerosis OR dorsal spine
CO	casualty officer		**DT**	delirium tremens
C/O	complains of		**DTP**	diphtheria, tetanus and pertussis
COHSE	Confederation of Health Service Employees		**DT/Vac**	diphtheria and tetanus vaccine
COP	change of plaster		**DU**	duodenal ulcer
CS	cervical spine		**DV**	domiciliary visit
CSF	cerebrospinal fluid		**D & V**	diarrhoea and vomiting
CSU	catheter urine specimen		**DVT**	deep vein thrombosis
CT	coronary thrombosis		**DXT**	deep X-ray radiation therapy
CV	cardiovascular		**EBS**	emergency bed service
CVA	cerebrovascular accident OR cardiovascular accident		**ECG**	electrocardiogram
			ECT	electroconvulsive therapy
CVP	central venous pressure		**EDD**	expected date of delivery
CVS	cardiovascular system OR cerebrovascular system		**EEG**	electroencephalogram
			ENT	ear, nose and throat
Cx	cervix		**ESN**	educationally subnormal
CXR	chest X-ray		**ESR**	erythrocyte sedimentation rate
D & C	dilatation and curettage			
D & D	drunk and disorderly		**EUA**	examination under anaesthetic
DDA	Dangerous Drugs Act			

F	Fahrenheit	**GU**	gastric ulcer OR genito-urinary
FB	foreign body	**GUT**	genito-urinary tract
FH	foetal heart	**Gyn**	gynaecology
FHA	Fellow of the Institute of Health Service Administrators	**Hb**	haemoglobin
		HBP	high blood pressure
FHH	foetal heart heard	**HEC**	Health Education Council
FHNH	foetal heart not heard		
Fib	fibula	**HO**	house officer
FIMLT	Fellow of the Institute of Medical Laboratory Technology	**HP**	house physician
		HS	house surgeon OR heart sounds
FMF	foetal movement felt	**Ht**	height OR heart
FMP	first menstrual period	**ID**	infectious disease
FP	food poisoning	**IM**	intramuscular
FPA	Family Planning Association	**IOFB**	intraocular foreign body
FPC	Family Practitioner Committee OR Family Planning Clinic	**IQ**	intelligence quotient
		ISQ	in status quo (no change)
FT	full-term	**IU**	international unit
FTND	full-term normal delivery	**IUCD**	intra-uterine contraceptive device
GA	general anaesthetic	**IUD**	intra-uterine death OR intra-uterine device
GB	gall bladder		
GIT	gastro-intestinal tract	**IV**	intravenous
GMC	General Medical Council	**IVP**	intravenous pyelogram
GNC	General Nursing Council	**IZS**	insulin zinc suspension
GOC	General Optical Council	**JHDA**	Junior Hospital Doctors Association
GOK	God only knows		
GOT	glutamic oxaloacetic transaminase	**L**	left OR litre
		LA	local anaesthetic OR left atrium OR local authority OR left axilla
GP	general practitioner		
GPI	general paralysis of the insane		
GPT	glutamic pyruvic transaminase	**Lab**	laboratory
		LBP	low back pain
GTT	glucose tolerance test	**LDH**	lactic dehydrogenase

LE cells	lupus erythematosus cells		**MPU**	Medical Practitioners Union
LHA	local health authority OR Licentiate of the Institute of Health Service Administrators		**MR**	manual removal
			MRC	Medical Research Council
LIF	left iliac fossa		**MRU**	mass radiography unit
LIH	left inguinal hernia		**MS**	multiple sclerosis OR mitral stenosis OR musculo-skeletal
LLL	left lower lobe			
LMC	local medical committee		**MSU**	mid stream urine
LMN	lower motorneurone		**MXR**	mass X-ray
LMP	last menstrual period		**NAD**	no abnormality detected
LP	lumbar puncture			
LRTI	lower respiratory tract infection		**NBI**	no bony injury
			NBTS	National Blood Transfusion Service
LS	lumbar spine OR locomotor system		**ND**	normal delivery OR nervous disability OR not diagnosed
LV	lumbar vertebra OR left ventricle			
LVF	left ventricular failure		**NHS**	National Health Service
LVH	left ventricular hypertrophy		**NI**	national insurance
			NK	not known
MCD	mean corpuscular diameter		**NP**	nomen proprium (proper name)
MCH	mean corpuscular haemoglobin		**NPU**	not passed urine
			NS	nervous system
MD	mentally deficient OR muscular dystrophy OR medical doctor		**N & V**	nausea and vomiting
			OA	osteoarthritis
			OE	on examination OR oritis externa
MDU	Medical Defence Union			
MI	myocardial infarction OR mitral incompetence		**OHE**	Office of Health Economics
			OM	otitis media OR osteomyelitis
MMR	mass miniature radiography			
			Op	operation
MO	medical officer		**PA**	pernicious anaemia OR pressure area OR postero-anterior
MOH	medical officer of health			
MOP	medical out-patient			

331

Paed paediatric (relating to children)

Para number of times a woman has been pregnant (includes abortions as well as live children)

PBI protein bound iodine

PBZ phenylbutazone

PDS patent ductus arteriosus

PET pre-eclamptic toxaemia

PID prolapsed intravertebral disc

PM post mortem

PMB post-menopausal bleeding

PMH previous medical history

PN post-natal

PND paroxysmal nocturnal dyspnoea

PO post-operative

POP plaster of Paris

POSSUM patient operated selector mechanism

PP private patient

PPH post partum haemorrhage

PPP Private Patients Plan

PR per rectum

Prem premature

PS pulmonary stenosis

PT pulmonary tuberculosis

PTA prior to admission

PU passed urine OR peptic ulcer

PUO pyrexia of unknown origin

PV per vaginam

PZI protamine zinc insulin

R recipe (shorthand used at the start of prescriptions to mean 'take')

RA rheumatoid arthritis OR right atrium OR right axilla

RBC red blood corpuscles

RCM Royal College of Midwives

RCN Royal College of Nursing

Rh rhesus factor OR rheumatism

RHA Regional Health Authority

RIF right iliac fossa

RIH right inguinal hernia

RLL right lower lobe

RMO resident medical officer OR regional medical officer

RNO regional nursing officer

RS respiratory system

RSM Royal Society of Medicine

RSO resident surgical officer

RTA road traffic accident

RTI respiratory tract infection

RVH right ventricular hypertrophy

SB stillborn

SBE subacute bacterial endocarditis

SI system internationale OR sacro-iliac OR soluble insulin

SMO senior medical officer

SMR sub-mucous resection

SN	student nurse		**UTI**	urinary tract infection
SOB	short of breath		**V**	visit
SOP	surgical out-patient		**V7**	visit in seven days
ST	sanitary towel		**Vac**	vaccination
Staff	staff nurse		**VD**	venereal disease
SW	social worker		**VE**	vaginal examination
SWD	short wave diathermy		**VI**	virgo intacta (virginal)
T & A	tonsils and adenoids		**VP**	venous pressure
TAB	typhoid, paratyphoid A and B vaccine		**VSD**	ventricular septal defect
			VU	varicose ulcer
TAB/Chol	typhoid, paratyphoid A and B vaccine with cholera vaccine		**VV**	varicose vein
			Vx	vertex
TABT	typhoid, paratyphoid A and B vaccine with tetanus toxoid		**WBC**	white blood count
			WC	whooping cough
			WHO	World Health Organization
TB	tuberculosis			
Tet	tetanus		**WR**	Wasserman reaction
TLC	tender, loving care		**XR**	X-ray
TPR	temperature, pulse and respiration		**YOB**	year of birth
			Yr	year
TR	temporary resident			
TS	thoracic spine			
TT	tetanus toxoid OR tuberculin tested			

MISCELLANEOUS SYMBOLS

TV	trichomonas vaginalis
UMN	upper motor neurone
URTI	upper respiratory tract infection

2C7	to see in seven days
⌗	fracture
△	diagnosis
∏	menstrual period

A to Z directory of qualifications by abbreviation

Most of the generally recognized qualifications attained by health professionals can be summarized with the aid of abbreviations. These often appear after an individual's name. It is perhaps important to point out that a number of organizations, institutions and colleges award qualifications which are not generally recognized as being of value.

Members and fellows of colleges sometimes add a few letters when abbreviating their qualifications to tell the world where they studied and passed the necessary examinations. So, for example, the letters Lond, Edin and Irel denote that the accompanying qualification was obtained in London, Edinburgh or Ireland.

BAO Bachelor of the Art of Obstetrics

BCh Bachelor of Surgery

BChD Bachelor of Dental Surgery

BDS Bachelor of Dental Surgery

BM Bachelor of Medicine

BS Bachelor of Surgery

BSc Bachelor of Science

ChB Bachelor of Surgery

ChM Master of Surgery

CMB Certificated by Central Midwives' Board

DA Diploma in Anaesthetics

DAP & E Diploma in Applied Parasitology and Entomology

DCH Diploma in Child Health

DCMT Diploma in Clinical Medicine of the Tropics

DCP Diploma in Clinical Pathology

DCPath Diploma of the College of Pathologists

DDS Doctor of Dental Surgery

DFHom Diploma of the Faculty of Homoeopathy

DIH Diploma in Industrial Health

DLO Diploma in Laryngology and Otology

DM Doctor of Medicine

DMJ Diploma in Medical Jurisprudence

DMR(D) Diploma in Medical Radiology (Diagnosis)

DMR(T) Diploma in Medical Radiology (Therapy)

DMSA Diploma of Medical Services Administration

DN Diploma in Nutrition

DO Diploma in Ophthalmology

DObstRCOG Diploma in Obstetrics of the Royal College of Obstetricians and Gynaecologists

DPath Diploma in Pathology

DPH Diploma in Public Health

DPhysMed Diploma in Physical Medicine

DPM Diploma in Psychological Medicine

DRCPath Diploma of the Royal College of Pathologists

DSc Doctor of Science

DTM & H Diploma in Tropical Medicine and Hygiene

FBOA Fellow of the British Optical Association

FFARCS Fellow of the Faculty of Anaesthetists, Royal College of Surgeons

FFCM Fellow of the Faculty of Community Medicine

FFHom Fellow of the Faculty of Homoeopathy

FFRRCS Fellow of the Faculty of Radiologists, Royal College of Surgeons

FPS Fellow of the Pharmaceutical Society

FRCGP Fellow of the Royal College of General Practitioners

FRCP Fellow of the Royal College of Physicians

FRCPsych Fellow of the Royal College of Psychiatrists

FRCS Fellow of the Royal College of Surgeons

HVCert Certificate of the Council for the Education and Training of Health Visitors

LAHDubl Licentiate of Apothecaries Hall, Dublin

LCPS Licentiate of the College of Physicians and Surgeons

LDS Licentiate in Dental Surgery

LM Licentiate in Midwifery

LMRCPIrel Licentiate in Midwifery of the Royal College of Physicians of Ireland

LMRCSIrel Licentiate in Midwifery of the Royal College of Surgeons in Ireland

LMSSA Licentiate in Medicine and Surgery of the Society of Apothecaries of London

LRCP Licentiate of the Royal College of Physicians

LRCPS Licentiate of the Royal College of Physicians and Surgeons

LRCS Licentiate of the Royal College of Surgeons

LSA Licentiate of the Society of Apothecaries

LTM Licentiate in Tropical Medicine

MAO	Master of the Art of Obstetrics		**MRCGP**	Member of the Royal College of General Practitioners
MB	Bachelor of Medicine		**MRCOG**	Member of the Royal College of Obstetricians and Gynaecologists
MCh	Master of Surgery			
MChD	Master of Dental Surgery			
MChir	Master of Surgery		**MRCP**	Member of the Royal College of Physicians
MChOrth	Master of Orthopaedic Surgery			
MCPath	Member of the College of Pathologists		**MRCPath**	Member of the Royal College of Pathologists
MD	Doctor of Medicine		**MRCS**	Member of the Royal College of Surgeons
MFCM	Member of the Faculty of Community Medicine		**MS**	Master of Surgery
			MSc	Master of Science
MFHom	Member of the Faculty of Homoeopathy		**PhD**	Doctor of Philosophy
MPhil	Master of Philosophy		**RMN**	Registered Mental Nurse
MPS	Member of the Pharmaceutical Society		**SCM**	State Certified Midwife
			SEN	State Enrolled Nurse
MRad	Master of Radiology (Diagnosis and Therapy)		**SRN**	State Registered Nurse

Organ donors

Individuals who would like their organs to be used by transplant surgeons after they have died can obtain multi-organ donor cards either from their own general practitioner or from the DHSS Leaflets Unit, PO Box 21, Stanmore, Middlesex HA7 1AY.

Twelve million plastic donor cards were printed in the summer of 1981 and distributed through family doctors, chemists and the Royal National Institute for the Blind.

The wording on the card is 'I request after my death (a) that my kidneys/eyes/heart/liver/pancreas be used for transplantation or (b) any part of my body be used for the treatment of others'. The Medic Alert Foundation (see below) makes a special necklet engraved to show that the wearer is prepared to donate one or more of his or her organs.

Medic Alert

Today several million people around the world wear necklaces and bracelets carrying information about their medical conditions. Such items of jewellery are invaluable for individuals suffering from such disorders as epilepsy, drug sensitivity, diabetes and so on, since they provide any medical practitioner with immediately available information. People wearing Medic Alert bracelets and necklaces may also leave a more comprehensive account of their illness with a permanently manned office, the telephone number of which will also appear on the bracelet or necklace. The Medic Alert scheme is particularly suitable for travellers (address on p. 179).

Individuals who have a medical history short enough to be written on a modest sized piece of paper might invest in one of the commercially available devices such as the Medi-Gen Information Capsule or the SOS Talisman.

Guide to information sources

Information on medical topics is not difficult to find. There are a number of ways in which the interested reader can learn more about general health care or specific problems.

For those looking for advice and information about the health service the Department of Health and Social Security and Her Majesty's Stationery Office are the best sources.

The DHSS publishes a wide range of free leaflets which are intended to provide patients with an introduction to the services available. The 'Catalogue of social security leaflets' (NI 146) contains details of leaflets describing the wide variety of benefits payable to the sick, injured, retired, widowed etc. The catalogue and the individual leaflets can either be obtained from local social security offices or by writing to the DHSS Leaflets Unit (address p. 337).

For those whose need is for medical care rather than financial assistance the DHSS publishes a booklet entitled 'Help for handicapped people' (HB1) which can also be obtained from the address in Stanmore.

If you want leaflets describing the social security and medical care arrangements with other countries, the two most useful publications are 'Medical treatment during visits abroad' (SA 30) and 'Notice to travellers: health protection' (SA 35).

Her Majesty's Stationery Office publishes an ever-increasing number of leaflets, booklets, brochures and books on health service and health care topics. A catalogue of the publications available can be obtained from any government bookshop and the publications themselves can either be ordered through government bookshops or ordinary commercial bookshops. The government bookshop in London is at 49 High Holborn, London WC1V 6HB.

The Health Education Council also publishes a number of useful leaflets and brochures, many of which can be obtained without charge from the HEC at 78 New Oxford Street,

London WC1A 1AH. The Council publishes a catalogue which lists its own leaflets and in addition has a library of reference books and audio-visual material which it makes available to anyone interested.

In addition to these official publications there is, of course, no shortage of commercial publications dealing with medical topics. During 1980 the 'organ of the book trade', *The Bookseller*, reported that there were over 3300 new books published dealing exclusively with medical subjects. Most local bookshops and libraries stock a wide range of guide and reference books.

Those interested in the general history of medicine should look out for the classic guide *History of Medicine* by Fielding H. Garrison (published by Saunders). Among the most readable books on human anatomy and physiology are *The Wisdom of the Body* by W. B. Cannon (published by Norton) and *The Body in Question* by Jonathan Miller (published by Cape). Readers looking for more formal sources of information should try one or two of the many texts produced specifically for nurses.

Those intending to travel abroad and visit places in tropical countries off the beaten track can do no better than buy a small publication entitled *Preservation of Personal Health in Warm Climates* which is published by the Ross Institute of Tropical Hygiene at the London School of Hygiene and Tropical Medicine, Keppel Street (Gower Street), London WC1E 7HT.

The World Health Organization publishes a booklet entitled *Vaccination Certificate Requirements for International Travel and Health Advice to Travellers*. This contains a good deal of useful, practical advice in addition to information about legal requirements.

Many good pharmacology textbooks exist but the biggest and best is probably *Martindale: The Extra Pharmacopoeia* (published by the Pharmaceutical Press) which is currently in its 27th edition. *The British National Formulary* (published by the British Medical Association and the Pharmaceutical Society of Great Britain) is the text favoured by most practising doctors looking for information about drugs to prescribe but is available on general sale. My own book *The Home Pharmacy* (published by Pan in paperback) deals exclusively with those products which can be bought over the chemist's counter without a prescription. Readers looking for a searching analysis of the pharmaceutical industry and the world of drugs in general may be interested in *The Medicine Men* (published by Arrow as a paperback) which is, I am afraid, also one of my own books.

Of the many journals and magazines dealing exclusively with medical matters the only one that I know of that is free of drug company advertising (and therefore free of any suggestion that it may be subject to commercial pressures in selecting its editorial matter) is the *Drug and Therapeutics Bulletin* which is published by the Consumers' Association and is available to the general public through the Subscription Department, Consumers' Association, Caxton Hill, Hertford SG13 7LZ.

Very many drug companies themselves publish leaflets and booklets designed to provide patients with information about specific disease processes. Obviously these publications are often geared to fit in with the particular company's own marketing programme (a company making a drug intended for use in the treatment of high blood pressure is not likely to produce a booklet extolling the virtues of relaxation therapy). Nevertheless many of the publications are worth studying. General practitioners usually have access to these leaflets and will be happy to pass on any publications that they regard as useful.

Finally, it is worth remembering that nearly all the organizations and associations listed elsewhere in this book publish literature of one sort or another which they are happy to send to enquiring readers.

Index

This index can be used as an alternative to the contents pages to find your way around the book. General entries that will be useful in this way are picked out in **bold** type.

For professional and voluntary organizations see pp. 166–71 and 174–84.
For drug names see pp. 222–67.
For drug companies see pp. 285–94.
For abbreviations see pp. 328–36.

Page numbers in *italic* indicate key references.

abbreviations: used in medicine, *328–33*; of medical qualifications, *334–6*
abortion, 57, *81–2*, 108, 175; and British Pregnancy Advisory Service, 82; and National Health Service, 81; *and see* private and voluntary organizations
abreaction, *301*
accidents *see* emergencies
achillorraphy, *295*
acupuncture, *135*; *and see* statutory and professional organizations
adenectomy, *295*
adenoidectomy, *295*
adipectomy, *295*
adoption: medical report, 69; *and see* private and voluntary organizations
adrenalectomy, *295*
adrenaline, *268*
adrenocorticotropic hormone (ACTH), *268*
aerosol, *280*
alcoholism *see* private and voluntary organizations
Alexander Method, Principle or Technique, *135*
allergies to drugs, 276, 277; *and see* drugs, allergy reactions to

alternative medicine, *133–40*, 321; practitioners' qualifications, *140*
aluminium hydroxide *see* drugs; home medicines
alveolotomy, *295*
ambulance service, 23, 144
amniocentesis, 23, 82, *186*
amniotomy, *295*
amputation, *295*
anaemia *see* haematologist
anaesthetic, 112, *280*
anaesthetist, *122*
analgesic, *280*
anastomosis, *295*
aneurysmectomy, *295*
angiectomy, *295*
annuloplasty, *295*
anorectic, *280*
antacids, *280*; *and see* drugs
ante-natal care, 42, 51
antibiotics, 110, 198, 271, *280*; *and see* drugs
anticholinergic, *280*
anti-emetic, *280*
antihistamine, *280*; *and see* drugs
anti-infective, *280*; *and see* drugs
anti-inflammatory, *280*; *and see* drugs

For drug names A to Z see pp. 222–67

antiperspirant, *280*
antipyretic, *280*
antiseptic, *280*
antispasmodic, *280*
antrectomy, *295*
anxiolytic, *281*
aortotomy, *295*
aperient, *281*
apicectomy, *295*
aponeurectomy, *295*
apophysectomy, *296*
appendectomy, *296*
appendicectomy, *296*
application, *281*
appointments: with a GP, *58–63*; with
a hospital consultant, 149
apronectomy, *296*
Area Health Authorities, 18, 25; *and see*
National Health Service
arteriography, *186*
arterioplasty, *296*
arthritis *see* orthopaedic surgeon; private
and voluntary organizations
arthrodesis, *296*
artificial insemination, *83*
aspiration, *296*
aspirin, 137, 211, 307; *and see* drugs
associations: patients' *see* private and
voluntary organizations; professional
see statutory and professional organizations
asthma *see* private and voluntary organizations
astringent, *281*
attendance allowance *see* social security
benefits
audiology technicians, 131
audiometry, *186*
autopsy, *296*
avulsion, *296*

back pain *see* private and voluntary
organizations
balm, *281*
barbiturates, 214; *and see* drugs
barium enema examination, *187*
barium meal examination, 45, *186–7*
baths and bathing, *136*
biochemistry (alternative medicine treatment), *136*
biochemistry (branch of science), *187*

biofeedback, *136*
biopsy, 187, *296*
bladder, disorders of, 62; *and see* urologist
blepharectomy, *296*
block, *296*
blood, study of *see* haematologist; haema-
tology
blood pressure: and the contraceptive
pill, 271, 272; checks, 164, 272; disorders, 57, 62, 206, 211
blood samples, 128
blood tests, 45, *187*, 192
brain surgery, 126; *see also* neurosurgeon
breastfeeding: drugs during, *209*; and
oral contraceptives, *271*
breasts: screening, 187; tenderness of
see oral contraceptives; X-raying of
see mammography
breech, *296*
British associations: of patients *see* private and voluntary organizations; of
professionals *see* statutory and professional organizations
British Medical Association, 100, 167,
200, 339; booklets, 305, 307
British National Formulary, 200
British United Provident Association
(BUPA), 27, 31, 163, 318, 320
bronchoscopy, *187*, 190, *296*
Brook clinics *see* private and voluntary
organizations
bunionectomy, *296*
burrholes, *296*
bypass, *296*

Caesarian section *see* Cesarian section
calamine lotion *see* drugs; home medicines
cancer, 57; testing kits, 304; diagnosis
and treatment of *see* oncologist; radiotherapist; patients' associations *see*
private and voluntary organizations
capsule, *281*
capsulectomy, *296*
cardiac catheterization, *188*
cardiac function, *188*
cardiologist, *122*
cardiomyotomy, *296*
cartilage problems *see* orthopaedic surgeon

castration, *296*

casualty department, 45, 124, 143, 144, 145

cataracts *see* ophthalmologist

cathartic, *281*

caustic, *281*

cauterization, *296*

cephalotomy, *296*

certificate of confinement, 68

certificate of expected confinement, 68, 313

cervical smears, 164, *188*

Cesarian section, *296*

changing your doctor, *73–6,* 78

charitable organizations *see* private and voluntary organizations

chemosurgery, *296*

chest trouble, 62; *and see* private and voluntary organizations

child benefit *see* social security benefits

child care *see* private and voluntary organizations

child minders, licensing of, 131

child psychiatrist, 122

childbirth, 307; *and see* private and voluntary organizations

chiropodists, 40, 84, *127; and see* statutory and professional organizations

child's special allowance *see* social security benefits

chiropractic, *136; and see* statutory and professional organizations

cholangiostomy, *296*

cholecystectomy, *296*

cholecystography, *188*

chondrectomy, *296*

choosing your doctor, *70–73,* 78

circumcision, *296*

Citizens Rights Office, 177

clinical physiologist, *122*

clinics: ante-natal, 41; screening, *163–4;* VD, *148*

clipping, *296*

clitoridectomy, *296*

clitoridotomy, *296*

closure, *296*

colectomy, *297*

colitis, 128

collodion, *281*

colonoscopy, *188*

colorrhaphy, *297*

colostomy, 205, *297; and see* private and voluntary organizations

colpectomy, *297*

colporrhaphy, *297*

colposcopy, *189*

Committee on Safety of Medicines, 168, 208, 212, 216

Community Health Councils, 18, 20, 121

community health physician, 122

complaints: about GPs, *98–110;* about dentists, opticians and pharmacists, 102; about hospital doctors, specialists and hospital administration, *118–21;* about nurses, 103

computerized tomography, *189*

confidentiality, *83–7*

confusion *see* drugs, side effects of; home screening

consent, *87–8;* and 1959 Mental Health Act, 88, 148

constipation, 62; *and see* drugs, side effects of

consultant specialists, 113–15, 149, 156; and home visits, 114, 145

Consumers' Association: health publications, 326, 341

contraception: advising on, 68, *88–90,* 96, 97; oral, 96, 198, 207, *269–72;* sterilization, *97,* 300; *and see* private and voluntary organizations

convulsions: and measles vaccination, 275; and whooping cough vaccination, 277

coronary care unit, 144

coroner, 324, 325

corticosteroids: hormones, *268; and see* drugs

cosmetic surgery, 47, 125, *297,* 321

cottage hospitals, 41, 147

cough medicines, 207, 281; *and see* drugs

coughs, 62

craniectomy, *297*

craniotomy, *297*

cream, 204, *281*

cricoidectomy, *297*

For drug names A to Z see pp. 222–67

criminal injuries compensation *see* social security benefits
Criminal Injuries Compensation Board, 317
Crohn's disease, 123
cryptorchidopexy, *297*
curettage, *297*
cystectomy, *297*
cystitis, 62; *and see* private and voluntary organizations
cytoscopy, *189*

D and C, *297*
day case units, *146–7*
deafness *see* private and voluntary organizations
death certificate, 40, *68*, 135, *324*, *325*
death grant *see* social security benefits
deaths, 57; what to do when someone dies, *324–5*
debridement, *297*
decompression, *297*
decongestant, *281*
defibrillation, *297*
denervation, *297*
dental hygienists, 128
dental nurses, 128
dental therapists, 128
dentists, 40, *127–8*; complaints about, *102*
deodorant, *281*
Department of Health and Social Security, *16–17*, 19, 25, 101, 131, *168*, 199, *310*; and advice to travellers, 322; HM Inspector of Anatomy, 326; leaflets, *311*, *315*, *326*, *337*, *338*; and National Health Service, *17*, 19, 24, 311; and Personal Social Services, 16, 17, 19, *131*; and social security services, *16*, *131*, *310*
depression: after bereavement, 326; *and see* mental health care; private and voluntary organizations
dermatologist, *122*
'Dial a doctor', 32
diarrhoea, 62; while taking oral contraceptives, 270; and polio vaccination, 276; *and see* drugs, side effects of
dialysis, *297*
diatetics, *136*
diathermy, *297*

dieticians, *128*
digitalis, 137
dilation, *297*
Director of Social Services *see* Social Services
Directory of Private Hospitals and Health Services, 156, 158–9
disabled people's associations *see* private and voluntary organizations
disablement benefit *see* social security benefits
disarticulation, *297*
Disciplinary Committee (of General Medical Council) *see* Professional Conduct Committee
disinfectant, *281*
dispensing opticians, *130*
District Management Teams, *18*, 20, 25, 119
district nurses, *50*, 90, 146
diuretic, *282*; *and see* drugs
divertisulectomy, *297*
divine healing, *139*
dizziness *see* drugs, side effects of
donor schemes, *337*
drainage, *297*
drip-feeding, *151*, *153*
drowsiness *see* drugs, side effects of
drug companies, *285–94*
drugs, *196–267*; addiction to, 214 *and see* private and voluntary organizations; allergy reactions to, 211, 212, 213, 276, 277; branded and generic, 198–9; and breastfeeding, 209; for children, 209–10; controlled, 197; efficiency of, 199–200; forms in which prescribed, 203, 204, 223, 225–67; interaction between, 214; overdosage, 203; placebos, 200–201; poisoning, 214–15; and pregnancy, 208; prescriptions, 196–7, 204–206, 217–21; side effects of, 210–13, 224; storage of, 204; 'top ten' prescription groups, 207; uses of, 224, 225–67; way in which taken, 201
duodenectomy, *297*
dusting powder, *282*
dyslexia *see* private and voluntary organizations

ear, nose and throat (ENT) surgeon, 46, *122*

ECG (electrocardiography) technicians, 131
ECT *see* electroconvulsive therapy
eczema: and whooping cough vaccination, 277
EEG (electroencephalography) technicians, 131
electrocardiogram, 188
electrocardiography (ECG), *189*
electroconvulsive therapy (ECT), 117, *301*
electroencephalography (EEG), *189*
elixir, *282*
embolectomy, *297*
embrocation, *282*
emergencies: casualty department, 45, 143, 144, 145, 214; referrals to NHS hospitals, *43*, *143–4*; referrals to private hospitals, 157
emollient, *282*
emulsion, *282*
encephalography *see* ventriculography
endarterectomy, *297*
endocrinologist, *122*
endoscopy, *190*
enemas, 151, *282*
enterocolostomy, *297*
enucleation, *298*
epididymectomy, *298*
epilepsy: and measles vaccination, 275; and Medic Alert, 337; and whooping cough vaccination, 277; *and see* private and voluntary organizations
episiotomy, *298*
equipment for the disabled *see* private and voluntary organizations
ethics, medical: and the GP, *79–98*; and hospital specialists, *117–18*
euthanasia, *91–2*
evacuation, *298*
evisceration, *298*
evulsion, *298*
excision, *298*
expectorant, *282*
exploration, *298*
exposure, *298*
extraction, *298*
eye donors *see* donor schemes

eye specialist *see* ophthalmologist

fainting *see* drugs, side effects of
faith healing, *139*
family doctors *see* general practitioners
family income supplement *see* social security benefits
Family Planning Association 178
family planning clinics, 90
Family Practitioner Committees (FPCs), 20, 67, 69, 121; and choosing your GP, 70, 74; and changing your GP, 75; complaints to, *100–104*, 128; and dentists, 127–8; the GP's contract with, *34–5*, 37, 77, 99
fasciectomy, *298*
fenestration, *298*
follicle stimulating hormone (FSH), *268*
forensic pathologist, *123*
forensic psychiatrist, *123*
forms and certificates, *67–9*
fusion, *298*

gargle, *282*
gastrectomy, *298*
gastroenterologist, *123*
gastroscopy, *190*
gel, *282*
General Dental Council: and dentists, 127–8; and complaints to, 102; *and see* statutory and professional organizations
general hospitals *see* hospitals
General Medical Council, 31, 82–3, 91, 97–8, 119, 168; complaints to, 100, 104, *105–108*, 119; responsibilities of, 106; *and see* statutory and professional organizations
General Nursing Council, 129; complaints to, 103; *and see* statutory and professional organizations
General Optical Council, 130; complaints to, 102; *and see* statutory and professional organizations
general physician, 46, 125
general practitioner hospitals *see* hospitals

For drug names A to Z see pp. 222–67

general practitioners (GPs), *30–48*, *52–110*, 143; and appointments systems, 59–61, 63, 72; complaints about, *98–110*; and consultations, *58–66*; and deaths, 324–5; and Family Practitioner Committees, 20, *34–5*, 37, 67, 69, 70, 74, 75, 77, 99, *100–104*, 121, 127–8; and home visiting, 55, *58–9*, 60, 63, 103; and medical ethics, *79–98*; and the National Health Service, *32–40*; premises of, 40–41; and prescribing, 196–7, 215, *217–21*; and the primary care team, *48–52*; in private practice, *30–2*; professional status of, 70–1; referrals made by, *42–8*, 103, 111, 156; responsibilities of, *30*; and routine check-ups, 164; and side effects of drugs, 212–13; treatment provided by, 41–2; and vaccinations, 274

general surgeon, 46, 125
geriatric hospitals *see* hospitals
geriatrician, 46, *123*
germicide, *282*
glucagon, 268
glucose tolerance test (GTT), *196*
GPs *see* general practitioners
graft, *298*
granules, *282*
gravitonics, *137*
guardian's allowance *see* social security benefits
gynaecologist, *123*

haematologist, *123*
haemophilia *see* private and voluntary organizations
hallucination *see* drugs, side effects of
headache *see* drugs, side effects of
health centres, 40, 41
Health Education Council, 169, 187; publications, 305, 307, 322, *338–40*
health farms and hydros, 157
health insurance: against accidental injury, 14; private, 27, 31, *318–21*; statutory, *310–17*; travel, *322–3*
health services, administration of, *14–26*; *and see* Department of Health and Social Security; social security benefits; social services

Health Services Commissioner, 100, 120, 121
health visitors, 45, 48, 51, *129*; *and see* statutory and professional organizations
heart surgery, 126; *and see* cardiologist; operative procedures
hemorrhoidectomy, *298*
hepatectomy, *298*
herbalism, *137*
hermorrhaphy, *298*
holistic medicine, *137*
home care, *303–8*
home helps, 17, 52, *128*, 131
home medicines, *307–8*
home screening, *304–7*
homoeopathy, *137*; *and see* statutory and professional organizations
homosexuality *see* private and voluntary organizations
hormone producing glands, *268*; *and see* endocrinologist
hormones, *268*; tests, *190*; treatments, *268*; *and see* drugs; oral contraceptives
hospitals: admissions to, 144–7, 148, 149; casualty department, 45, 124, 143, 144, 145; GP, 147–8; general (NHS), *142–6*; geriatric, 142, 143, 147; hierarchy in, 112–13; maternity, 143; mental, 142; out-patients' department, 43, 54; private, 113, *155–7*; routines, 150–3; *and see* clinics; emergencies; health farms and hydros; investigations and tests; nursing homes; residential homes; operative procedures
hot flushes *see* drugs, side effects of
house officer, 112, 116
house surgeon, 112
hydrotherapy, *136*, 157
hymenectomy, *298*
hypnosis, *138*
hypnotic, *282*; *and see* drugs
hypophysectomy, *298*
hypopituitarism, 211
hypotensives, 211
hysterectomy, 65, *298*
hysterotomy, *298*

ilectomy, *298*
ileocolostomy, *298*

ileostomy, *298*; *and see* private and voluntary organizations
immunization *see* vaccination
implant, *298*
impotence *see* drugs, side effects of
incision, *298*
Independent Hospital Group Ltd, 156
indigestion, 62; *and see* drugs, side effects of; home medicines
induction, *298*
infant mortality, in Britain, 21, 22–23
information on medical topics, *338–40*
inhalation, *282*; *and see* home medicines
injection, *282*
injury benefit *see* social security benefits
inquest, 324, 325
Institute of Health Service Administrators, 169
instrument examination, *190*
insufflation, *282*
insulin, *268*
insurance *see* health insurance
intensive care unit, 144
intensive therapy unit, 144
intravenous feeding *see* drip-feeding
intravenous pyelography, *190*
intubation, *298*
intussusception reduction, *298*
invalid care *see* nursing homes; private and voluntary organizations
invalidity pension *see* social security benefits
investigations and tests, *186–94*
iridectomy, *298*

jejunedectomy, *298*
junior house physician, *112*
junior registrar, *112*

kaolin mixture *see* home medicines
keratolytic, *282*
kidney donors *see* donor schemes
kidneys *see* nephrologist; urologist

laminectomy, *299*
laparoscopy *see* peritoneoscopy
laparotomy, *191*, *299*

laryngectomy, *299*
lavage, *299*
laxative, *282*; *and see* drugs; home medicines
lesbianism *see* private and voluntary organizations
leucotomy, *299*
leukaemia *see* haemotologist; private and voluntary organizations
ligation, *299*
linctus, *283*
liniment, *283*
lipectomy, *299*
lithotomy, *299*
lobectomy, *299*
lotion, *283*, *284*
lozenge, *283*
lumbar puncture, *191*
lumpectomy, *299*
lung function, *191*
lymphadenectomy, *299*

mammography, *191*
mammoplasty, *299*
Manor House Hospital *see* health insurance, private
marriage guidance *see* private and voluntary organizations
mastectomy, *299*; *and see* private and voluntary organizations
mastoidectomy, *299*
maternity benefit *see* social security benefits
maternity hospitals, 143
Medic Alert Foundation, 213, *337*; *and see* private and voluntary organizations
medical associations *see* statutory and professional organizations
medical card (FP4), *67*; and registering with a GP, 73, 74; and the Family Practitioner Committee, 102
Medical Directory, 70, 71
medical ethics *see* ethics, medical
medical jargon *see* abbreviations used in medicine
medical laboratory technicians, *128*
Medical Register, 70, 107

For drug names A to Z see pp. 222–67

Medical Research Council, 85; *and see* statutory and professional organizations

Medical Services Committee, 101, 102

medicated, *283*

medicines *see* drugs; home medicines

Medicover, 32, 319

Medi-Gen Information Capsule, 337

meditation, *138*

meniscectomy, *299*

mental health care: hospitals, 142; involuntary admissions, 148; nurses, 129; psychiatrist, 125; psychiatry, 112; psychotherapist, 125; psychotherapy, 301; *and see* private and voluntary organizations

microscopy, *191*

midwives, 51, *129*

migraine *see* private and voluntary organizations

mixture, *283*

mobility allowance *see* social security benefits

morphine, 137; *and see* drugs

mortality, infant *see* infant mortality

mothers' organizations *see* private and voluntary organizations

mouthwash, *283*

multiple sclerosis *see* private and voluntary organizations

muscular dystrophy *see* private and voluntary organizations

music therapy, *138*

myectomy, *299*

myelography, *191*

myotomy, *299*

national associations of patients *see* private and voluntary organizations

national associations of professionals *see* statutory and professional organizations

National Health Service: and abortion, 81; administration of, *14–26*; and the EEC, 21, 322; and the GP, *32–40*; hospitals and clinics, 14, *142–53*, 320, 321; and prescriptions, 204–205; private consultants in, 321; private wards in, 155, 321; *vis à vis* private health care, 26–8; Reorganization Act 1974, 15, 22; residential homes, 153–4; and specialists, 111–15; and visitors to Britain, 323; and waiting lists, 145, 146, 150, 156

National Health Service Central Register, 188

nature cure, *138*

nausea *see* drugs, side effects of; oral contraceptives, side effects of

neomycin, allergy to *see* vaccination

nephrectomy, *299*

nephrologist, *123*

nervous system *see* neuroradiologist; neurosurgeon

neuroradiologist, *124*

neurosurgeon, *124*

non-contributory invalidity pension *see* social security benefits

noradrenalin, 268

nurses: district, *50*, 90, 146; midwife, *51*, *129*; practice, *50–1*, 84, 90; private, *132*; state enrolled, 50, *129*; state registered, 50, *129*; *and see* statutory and professional organizations

Nurses Agencies Act 1957, 132

nursing homes, *158–62*

Nursing Homes Act 1975, 159

obliteration, *299*

obstetrician, 42, 46, 51, *124*; *and see* gynaecologist

obstetrics, 112

occupational health specialist, *124*

occupational therapist, 51, *130*; *and see* statutory and professional organizations

occupational therapy, *301*

oesophagoscopy, *191*

oestrogen, *268*; *and see* oral contraceptives

ointment, 203, *283*

oncologist, *124*

oophorectomy, 299

operative procedures, *295–300*

ophthalmic optician *see* opticians

ophthalmic surgeon *see* opticians

ophthalmologist, 124

opticians: ophthalmic optician, *130*; ophthalmic surgeon, *130*; complaints about, 102; *and see* statutory and professional organizations oral contraceptives: advising on, 96; how to use them, *270–1*; side effects of, *271–2*; types of, *269–70*; *and see* drugs

orchidectomy, *299*

organ donors *see* donor schemes

organizations: for patients *see* private and voluntary organizations; for professionals *see* statutory and professional organizations

orthopaedic surgeon, 46, *124*

orthoptics, 130

orthoptist, *130*

ostectomy, *299*

osteoarthritis, 125

osteopathy, 136, *139*; *and see* statutory and professional organizations

osteotomy, *299*

otoplasty, *299*

out-patients *see* hospitals

oxytocin, allergy to *see* vaccination

pain killers, 197, 198, 207; *and see* drugs; home medicines

paint (medicated), *283*

palpitations *see* drugs, side effects of

pancreas *see* hormone producing glands

pancreatectomy, *299*

panhysterectomy, *299*

papillectomy, *299*

paracetamol *see* drugs; home medicines

parathyroidectomy, *299*

Parkinson's disease *see* private and voluntary organizations

paste, *283*

pathologist, *124*, 191, 325

pathology, *191*; laboratory, 193

patient participation, 78–9

patients' associations *see* private and voluntary organizations

patients' rights, *94–6*

peak flow meter, *192*

Penal Cases Committee (of General Medical Council) *see* Preliminary Proceedings Committee

peritoneoscopy, *192*

pessary, *283*

pharmaceutical companies *see* drug companies

pharmacist, 197, 202, 218; complaints about, 102

pharmacologist, *125*

phlebotomy, *299*

phrenology, *139*

physically handicapped, care for the *see* private and voluntary organizations

physician, *125*

physiotherapists, 51, *130*; *and see* statutory and professional organizations

physiotherapy, *301*

pill, *283*; contraceptive *see* oral contraceptives

placebos, 199, *200–1*

plastic surgeon, *125*

plastic surgery *see* operative procedures

pneumonectomy, *299*

polpectomy, *299*

polymixin, allergy to *see* vaccination

post mortem, 324, 325; *and see* pathologist; pathology

post-natal classes, 129

potion, *283*

poultice, *283*

powder, *283*

practice nurses, *50–1*, 84, 90

prastatectomy, *299*

pregnancy: advice on *see* private and voluntary organizations; ante-natal care, 42, 51; booklets on, 307, 338; drugs during, 208; home confinement, 96; GP and, 42; maternity hospitals and wards, 51, 143; midwife and, *51, 129*; obstetrician and, 42, 51, 124; post-natal care, 129; unplanned *see* private and voluntary organizations; urine test, 193; *and see* abortion; amniocentesis

Preliminary Proceedings Committee (of General Medical Council), 107–8

prescriptions, 31, 41, 135, *196*, 200, 202, 303; charges, 196, *204*; 'dog Latin' used in, 217–21; exemption from charges, 67, *204–5*, 316; reading, *217–21*; repeat, 205–8; 'top

For drug names A to Z see pp. 222–67

ten' prescription groups, *207*; *and see* drugs

preservative, *283*

private and voluntary organizations, *174–84*

private health care, *26–8*, 113; *Directory of Private Hospitals and Health Services*, 156, 158–9; and GPs, *30–32*; hospitals, 113, *155–7*; insurance, *318–21*; nurses, *132*; nursing homes, *158–62*; screening clinics, 32, *163–4*; specialists, *111–12*

Private Patients Plan (PPP), 27, 318, 320

proctologist, *125*

proctoscopy, *192*

Professional Conduct Committee (of General Medical Council), 107–108

progesterone, *268*; *and see* oral contraceptives

prolactin, *268*

prophylactic, *284*

psoriasis *see* private and voluntary organizations

psychiatric care: hospitals, 143; *and see* mental health care; private and voluntary organizations

psychiatrist, 46, *125*

psychiatry, 112

psychic surgery *see* spiritual healing

psychosurgery, 117

psychotherapist, *125*

psychotherapy, *301*

purgative, *284*

pyloroplasty, *299*

qualifications: alternative medicine, *140*; orthodox medicine, *334–6*

radiesthesia, *139*

radioactive isotopes test, *192*

radiographer, 125

radiologist, *125*, 186

radionics, *139*

radiotherapist, *125*

radiotherapy, *302*

rape *see* private and voluntary organizations

ray treatment *see* radiotherapist; X-rays

reduction, *299*

Regional Health Authorities, 17, 18, 25, 66, 119

Register of Approved Private Hospitals and Nursing Homes, *170*

Register of Medical Practitioners, 135

Registered Nursing Home Association, 158

Registered Rest Home Association, 158

remedial gymnasts, *130*

residential homes, 153–4

rest homes *see* nursing homes

retirement pension *see* social security benefits

revascularization, *299*

rheumatism *see* private and voluntary organizations

rheumatoid arthritis *see* rheumatologist

rheumatologist, *125*

rhinoplasty, *299*

rhytidectomy, *300*

Royal College of General Practitioners, 71; *and see* statutory and professional organizations

Royal colleges of professionals *see* statutory and professional organizations

rub, *284*

rubefacient, *284*

salpingo-oophorectomy, *300*

Salvation Army *see* private and voluntary organizations

Samaritans *see* private and voluntary organizations

saunas *see* baths and bathing

scanning *see* computerized tomography

schizophrenia *see* private and voluntary organizations

school dental service, *130–1*

school health officials, *130*

screening, *300*; clinics, 32, *163–4*; home, *304–6*

section, *300*

sedative, *284*

senior hospital administrator, 119

senior house officer (SHO), 112, 113

senior registrar, 112

sexual activity, changes in *see* oral contraceptives, side effects of

sexual organs, diseases of *see* venereologist

shake lotions, *284*

shunt, *300*

sick note, 39, 62, 67, 91, 103, 135

sickness benefit *see* social security benefits

side effects of drugs *see* drugs, side effects of

sigmoidoscopy, *192*

sinus problems *see* ear, nose and throat surgeon

sinusotomy, *300*

skin preparations, 204, 207, 224; *and see* drugs

skin rash *see* drugs, allergy reactions to; side effects of

sleeping pills, 203, 206, 207; in hospital, 150–1; *and see* drugs

social security benefits, 310, *311–17*; contributory: child's special allowance, *313*; death grant, *314*, 326; invalidity benefit, 312, *313*; maternity benefit, *313*; retirement pension, *314*; sickness benefit, 17, *312*; unemployment benefit, *312*; widow's benefit, *314*, 326; non-contributory: attendance allowance, *316*; child benefit, *315*, 317; criminal injuries compensation, *317*; family income supplement, *315–16*; guardian's allowance, *317*; injury benefit and disablement benefit, *315*; invalid care allowance, *316*; invalidity pension, *316–17*; mobility allowance, *316*; supplementary benefit, *316*; 'Which benefit?' leaflet, 311, 317

social services, local, 16, 131; *and see* Social Services

Social Services: Director of, 128, 154; Secretary of State for, 16, 131; Personal, 16, 17, 19, 131

social workers, 17, 48, 84, *131*, 154

Socialist Medical Association, 171

societies: for patients *see* private and voluntary organizations; for professionals *see* statutory and professional organizations

solution, *284*

SOS Talisman, 337

spastics *see* private and voluntary organizations

specialists, *42–8*, *111–26*, 127; in the National Health Service, *112–13*; private, *111–12*, 145, 155

speech therapists, 131; *and see* statutory and professional organizations

sphincterotomy, *300*

spina bifida *see* private and voluntary organizations

spinal injuries *see* private and voluntary organizations

spirit, *284*

spiritual healing, *139*

splenectomy, *300*

spray, *284*

Standing Conference on Drug Abuse, 184

stapedectomy, *300*

state benefits *see* social security benefits

state enrolled nurse (SEN), 50, *129*

state registered nurse (SRN), 50, *129*

statutory and professional organizations, *166–71*

sterilization, 97, *300*

steroids *see* drugs

stillbirths *see* private and voluntary organizations

stimulant, *284*

Sun Alliance Hospital Benefits Plan, 319

supplementary benefit *see* social security benefits

suppositories, 151, 203, *284*; *and see* drugs, forms in which prescribed

surgeon, 126; *and see* specialists

surgery (GP's) *see* general practitioners, consultations; premises of

surgery (operations) *see* operative procedures; specialists

suspension, *300*

suture, *300*

swab tests, *192*

sympathectomy, *300*

synovectomy, *300*

syphilis *see* VD clinics; venereologist

syringing, *300*

tablet, *284*; *and see* drugs

talisman therapy, *139*

For drug names A to Z see pp. 222–67

tap, *300*
tenotomy, *300*
tension *see* drugs, side effects of
termination, *300*
test meal, *193*
test tube babies *see* artificial insemination
testosterone, *268*
tests *see* investigations and tests
thalidomide *see* private and voluntary organizations
thermography, 193
thoracic surgeon, 126
thrombectomy, *300*
thyroid gland *see* hormone producing glands
thyroidectomy, *300*
tonsillectomy, *300*
tracheostomy, *300*
traction, *300*
tranquillizers *see* drugs
transfusion, *300*, *302*
transplantation, 23, *117*, *300*
transsexuals *see* private and voluntary organizations
tremors *see* drugs, side effects of
trusts *see* private and voluntary organizations

ultrasound, 23, *193*
unemployment benefit *see* social security benefits
ureterotomy, *300*
urine test, 39, 45, *128*, 164, *193*; *and see* pathology
urologist, 123, *126*

vaccination, *272–7*; certificates, 68, 276; when going abroad, *272–7*, 322; cholera, 273, *275*; diphtheria, 39, 272, *275*; infective hepatitis, *275*; influenza, *275*; measles, *275*; poliomyelitis, 272, 273, *276*; rubella, *276*; smallpox, 272, *276*; tetanus, 139, 273, *276*; tuberculosis, 228, 272, *276*; typhoid, *276*; whooping cough (pertussis), 39, 273, *277*; yellow fever, 277
vaginoplasty, *300*
vagotomy, *300*

valvotomy, *300*
vapour rub, *284*
vasectomy, 184, *300*
vasodilator, *284*
VD clinics, *148*
venereologist, 126, 148
venesection, *300*
venipuncture, *300*
venography, *194*
ventriculography, *194*
ventrosuspension, *300*
version, *300*
vitamins, 136, 207, *278–9*
voluntary organizations *see* private and voluntary organizations
vomiting: and the contraceptive pill, 270–1; and polio vaccine, 276; *and see* drugs, side effects of
vulvectomy, *300*

weight, body, changes in *see* oral contraceptives, side effects of; screening, home
weight problems *see* private and voluntary organizations
welfare state *see* National Health Service; social security benefits; social services
Western Provident Association (WPA), 27
wheezing *see* drugs, side effects of
widow's benefit *see* social security benefits
wind (flatulence) *see* drugs, side effects of
women's organizations *see* private and voluntary organizations
World Health Organization, 171, 198, 222–3, 339

xerography *see* X-rays
X-rays, 45, *194*; arteriography, *186*; barium enema examination, *187*; barium meal examination, *186*; cholecystography, *188*; mammography, *191*; myelography, *191*; neuroradiologist, *124*; radiologist, 125; radiotherapy, *306*; xerography, *194*

For drug names A to Z see pp. 222–67